Waking into "The Big O"

A New Look at
Sleep-Related Female Orgasms

By

Franceen King, Ph.D.

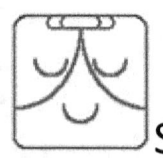Self-Awareness Publishing Co.
A Division of The Self-Awareness Institute
Lutz, FL 33559

ISBN-13: 978-1469942155

Publication date: June 6, 2012
Minor revisions: July 6, 2012

Additional copies may be obtained from:
www.franceenking.com
www.amazon.com

Correspondence: DrFranceen@aol.com

AUTHOR'S NOTE

This is my second book on the very neglected topic of Sleep-Related Female Orgasms (SRFOs). The first was a slight revision of my 2006 Doctoral Dissertation, originally submitted to the American Academy of Clinical Sexologists for a PhD in Clinical Sexology. I published it in book form in 2011 because there is almost nothing in print available to the public on this topic.

My first book, entitled **Sleep-Related Female Orgasms: A Survey of Biological, Psychological, Sociological and Cultural Factors,** covers a broad range of information, research data, and opinion about women's orgasms and female sexuality, throughout history, and is easily available from Amazon.com or my website.

This book, **Waking into "The Big O,"** is a follow-up and companion. It contains fascinating statistics regarding this phenomenon based on responses to an online survey, as well as commentary from women of all ages. Whether you are a woman or a man, this book is likely to forever change the ways you think about women's sexuality.

ACKNOWLEDGEMENTS

First and foremost, I want to acknowledge all of the women who took time to complete my lengthy online survey. This book would not be possible without their interest, motivation, commitment, courage, and candor. For this, I am extremely grateful. Collectively, they have made a huge contribution to the understanding of women's sexuality and sexual responses.

Secondly, I want to acknowledge Alfred C. Kinsey and his team of researchers for their curiosity and dedication. Without their work in the 1940s and 50s, almost nothing about this topic would be known.

I am grateful to all of the sexological researchers, clinicians, and educators who have followed in Kinsey's footsteps. I have cited the work of so many people in this and my previous book, looking for clues and perhaps wisdom.

Most authors thank their publishers and editors. Since this book is self-published and edited, I do not really have people in those roles to thank. Nonetheless, I do want to acknowledge Amazon.com for making self-publishing so easy and affordable through their subsidiary createspace.com. With their tools and distribution channels they have truly transformed opportunities for self-expression for people in so many different fields.

I want to thank all of my family, friends, professional colleagues, clients, and workshop participants who have shared their stories with me, encouraged me, or just listened to me "think out loud" about this topic or the challenges of putting words on paper. At the top of this list I put my husband, Raymond Schmidt, who has endured my occasional eccentricities, and provided a wide-range of day-to-day support for me as I have engaged this process.

Lastly, I thank the Goddess within us all, the feminine consciousness who desires a greater voice in this world of the 21st century.

ABOUT THE AUTHOR

As a Licensed Mental Health Counselor, Dr. Franceen King has had a clinical practice in Lutz, Florida, since 1981. Through her business, *The Self-Awareness Institute*, she has worked with individuals and couples in a counseling setting, and conducted workshops on a wide variety of topics throughout the state of Florida.

Since 1986, she has designed and conducted week-long residential workshops at *The Monroe Institute* in Virginia on topics related to consciousness expansion and exploration. She also conducts outreach workshops throughout the world, especially Japan. Her life-long interests in lucid dreaming and paranormal perception have led her to explore many different philosophies and disciplines.

She began her career in the Washington, D.C. area where she spent seven years at the National Institutes of Health as a management intern and employee development specialist, with focus on Executive Development and Organization Development. After leaving NIH, she formed training and consulting firm, *Spectrum Associates, Inc.*, which provided services to numerous government agencies.

After moving to Florida in 1980, she shifted the focus of her work from organizations to individuals. Since 1995, she has been an ordained minister in the *Church of the Creator* with special interest in spiritual healing modalities.

She received her B.A. degree (psychology) from Mary Washington College of the University of Virginia (now Mary Washington University), her M.A. degree (community mental health counseling) from Hood College in Frederick, MD, and her Ph.D. (clinical sexology) from the American Academy of Clinical Sexologists, now in Orlando, FL.

DEDICATION

This book is dedicated to all women,
in celebration of our bodies, minds, and Spirit!

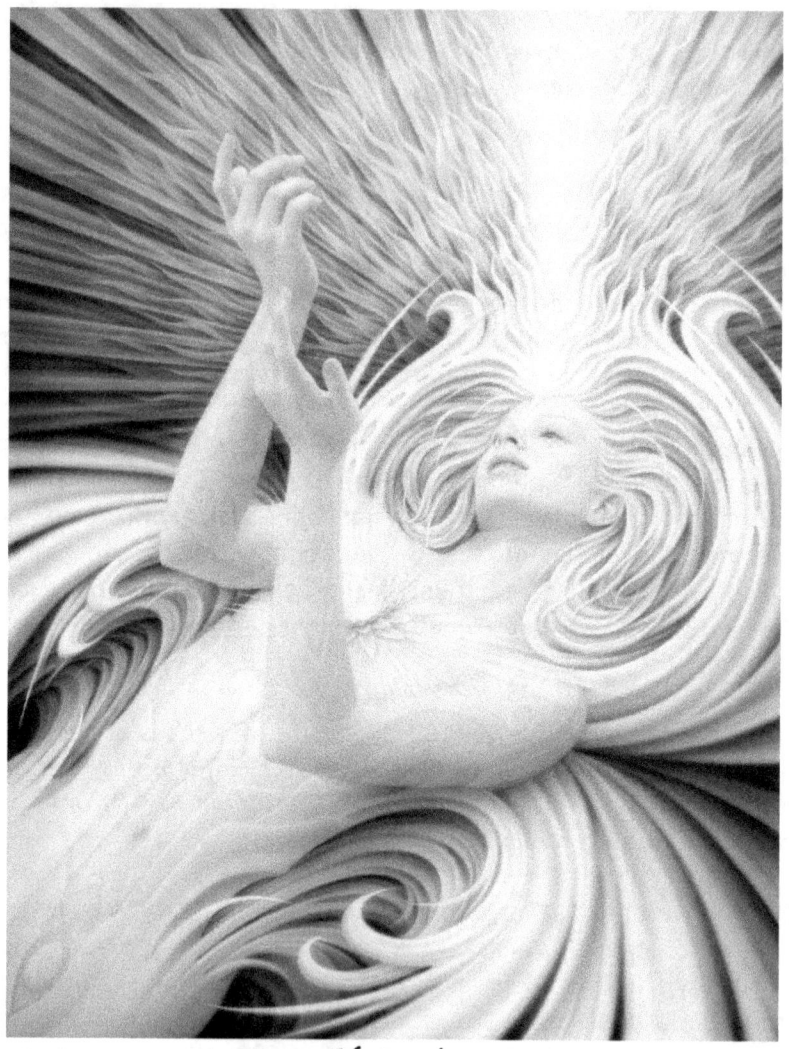

Yemanja
(The Awakening of the Heart)
With permission of the artist
A. Andrew Gonzalez
www.sublimatrix.com

TABLE OF CONTENTS

INTRODUCTION

Did *you* know that women are sometimes awakened from sleep by very physical, often very intense, orgasms? If this is news to you, you're not alone. My initial, informal surveys on this topic in 2004-5 indicated that approximately 70% of men, and almost 30% of women were not aware of this. Not all women experience these; but for those who do, they can sometimes be life-changing.

Sleep-Related Female Orgasms (SRFOs) are neither unhealthy nor rare. I've known about these sleep orgasms since I started experiencing them during my freshman year in college at age 17. My first experiences of these awakening orgasms would begin during a dream with some kind of vaguely romantic, sexual, or erotic content. (That's what allowed me to interpret these experiences as orgasms, rather than some kind of seizure!) I'd experience a rush of sexual arousal, the flushing, muscle tightness, and then as this peaked and released, the strong contractions in my vagina and pelvis would begin. These were very physical, and would wake me from the dream.

I did not know much about sex or orgasm at that time, but had heard that guys have "wet dreams." So I assumed my experiences meant that girls have something similar.
I do not recall discussing these with anyone, but over the years I would occasionally read brief comments that women sometimes have orgasms triggered by dreams. Usually this would be as an afterthought in an article about dreams, teen

1

boys, masturbation, or some other topic: "Some women have these too."

In any event, I assumed that these were normal...that I was normal. I was obviously healthy, and as I grew in sexual awareness and experience, I concluded that my range of sexual responsiveness was also healthy and normal.

Sometimes the dreams which preceded these orgasms did not seem to have anything obvious to do with sex, sensuality, desire, romance, or physical stimulation. And more rarely, sometimes I was not even aware of dreaming before these physical experiences began.

Regardless of why these might have happened, I considered my awakening orgasms to be pleasant surprises, and often hilariously funny when I looked at the dream content. Afterwards, I would feel great...and grateful! Today I am in my mid 60s. I've been with my husband for over 40 years now, and I still experience these.

Throughout my life I've worked with people in many emotionally intimate ways, primarily as a Licensed Mental Health Counselor in private practice, and as a group leader or facilitator conducting multi-day, residential, workshops related to a variety of personal growth topics.   I have often listened to reports and concerns about sexual feelings and behaviors. However, I don't recall anyone, male or female, ever mentioning or asking about these sleep-related orgasms until I began asking questions.

While working on a Ph.D. degree in Clinical Sexology during the 2004-5 periods, I began testing sample interview questions regarding a different topic. I noticed that several people began talking to me about their sleep-related orgasms, expressing worry or concern.   One woman mentioned that she had asked her male therapist about these and he replied that he had never heard of such a thing. Quite honestly, I was shocked. But as I began talking with some of my colleagues and workshop participants, I soon discovered that this lack of knowledge was not uncommon, even among health professionals. A lack of awareness and accurate information in the public domain can easily lead to worry and concern. It also provides opportunities for misunderstanding, self-doubt, and superstition.

It was this lack of general public awareness that prompted me to write my 2006 doctoral dissertation on this topic, essentially exploring the question, "Why don't more people know that women have sleep-related orgasms?" There are many reasons, including long-standing, erroneous, cultural beliefs and fears about women's sexuality. There are also some very current reasons for the lack of awareness. One is that this topic is not included in any sex education curricula that I could access. It is only rarely mentioned in books or magazine articles.

Another obvious reason for lack of pubic awareness is that this topic has been neglected in recent sexological research, although that has not been the case historically. Questions about sleep-related orgasms have not been included in any of the major surveys about human sexuality or sexual behavior since Alfred Kinsey's work in the late 1940s, and early 50s, published in 1953. It is a complex subject to study thoroughly because it spans several different fields including: sexology, sleep physiology, neurophysiology, endocrinology, psychology, consciousness, dreaming, anthropology, and spirituality.

It also brings the mind-body connection to the forefront, since these orgasms occur without any physical stimulation or sexual behavior. For most of the 20th century,

3

many of our social sciences, including psychology, focused on behavior. Only in recent years has it become once again more acceptable to study consciousness, the mind-body connection, or the role of thought and imagination.

In my dissertation, I pulled together all the information, opinion, statistics, research, and commentary I could find related to this topic, spanning many fields and much of human history.

Following completion of my dissertation, I posted the Abstract and Introduction online to provide information to the general public because there was so little available. In the years since then I have received numerous "thank-you" emails and letters from both women and men. Fortunately, the internet has made information about almost every topic more available...especially sex! I have noticed various blogs, as well as health and advice columns, citing or quoting from my postings.

Recently, for easier access, I decided to make that full dissertation available in book form titled, **Sleep-Related Female Orgasms: A Survey of Biological, Psychological, Sociological, and Cultural Factors**. It is filled with interesting information about female sexuality, most of which will not be repeated in this book. I've included the Table of Contents as Appendix A. The full book can be ordered from www.franceenking.com or www.Amazon.com. In cases where I excerpt sections from that book, I will put them in italics.

In late 2006, I also posted an internet survey to gather more current information regarding this response, and test some of the 29 possible research hypotheses which I identified. The survey is included as Appendix B – **A Research Survey of Sleep-Related Female Orgasms and Sex Dreams.**

4

This is a rather lengthy, detailed, technologically primitive survey. Knowing what I know now, I would probably change some of the questions. Nonetheless, many of the responses are enlightening and provide new information about this phenomenon. The responses also point to some new directions for further investigation of this topic.

This project has been on the "back burner" for me these past few years, due to other professional commitments and the slow pace at which survey responses have arrived. Nonetheless, I've learned a lot! My original intention when I began this survey was to write a scholarly journal article. Eventually I realized that the audience most in need of this information was the general public. Consequently, thanks to the ease of self-publishing, I have decided to present my findings from the survey responses in this book format. I consider this offering to be simply a beginning rather than any kind of final word. Perhaps it will arouse the curiosity of other researchers who might have the equipment, facilities, or other resources to explore this further.

I am profoundly grateful to all the women who took time to complete my survey and share their comments, questions, and experiences with me. So often, I have been moved by their honesty and touched by their desires to contribute to greater awareness regarding female sexuality. Most of the women who found and responded to my survey were women who had been experiencing sleep-related orgasms and consulted the internet for more information. Therefore, they are not a representative sample of all women. They are, however, the largest group of sleep orgasm experiencers that has been studied since the Kinsey Report published in 1953. They are the only group of healthy women above college that has been studied at all since then.

Needless to say, much has changed in our world during the past 60 years, both culturally and scientifically.

This book, *Waking into "The Big O,"* includes both statistics and commentary from my survey. The statistical data in this book comes from the first 200 responses, which include 174 sleep orgasm experiencers from ages 15 to 85. Because I think it is important to let women speak for themselves, I am including commentary from beyond the first 200 surveys as well as emails. Obviously, I have not been able to include every comment, but I probably will include more than many readers might like. I personally find every single comment to be interesting, and I have tried to include comments from women across the age span. I feel strongly that it is time for our culture to "get real" about female sexuality in general, and allow women a voice as fully embodied sexual beings.

If you would like to share about your experiences, the survey is still posted at www.franceenking.com/sexsurve.htm At some point in the future, I might publish a revised edition of this book with more data.

Although this book is intended primarily as a current overview for the general public, I hope that sex educators and researchers will also find it useful and, perhaps, even inspiring. Some of you might want to explore aspects of this subject in more scholarly depth by referring to my original work. Meanwhile, it is my hope that this book can provide assistance and re-assurance to both younger and older women, as well as their partners. It is also my hope that soon this topic will be included in every public school sex education class, and all training programs for health care providers.

Chapter 1

Lifting the Veils on Another Sex Secret

I cannot believe that in my entire life...that not one word of mention of any sort on this subject has ever been discussed in my presence or has come across to me in some kind of literature form! I'm so very disillusioned by this lack of knowledge about my own body and what it is so very capable of doing...How has something as large as this been tucked away from women???

I feel as though in this lifetime, this is the greatest inner personal discovery I may have ever made about myself and my inner body experience. I want to go on Oprah; I want to tell it out loud to Dr. Phil...to The View, etc. I want ALL women to know that this is possible and it is okay to talk about. What a wonderful subject to shed light on !!!
(survey participant, age 54, following a powerful SRFO)

It is 2012 as I write this, and it is hard to believe that there are any possible "sex secrets" given the abundance of sexual images and information in our culture today. Nonetheless, Sleep-Related Female Orgasms (SRFOs) seem to fall into this category. As mentioned in the Introduction, my informal surveys in the 2004-6 period suggested that almost

30 percent of women, and 70 percent of men, were unaware that such orgasms could occur.   I was even more surprised when I realized that many of the unaware were educated health care providers.   This lack of public awareness prompted me to research this topic for my 2006 PhD dissertation in Clinical Sexology.

As a culture, we have held so much of female sexuality in a shroud of mystery. Sometimes this mystery can enhance eroticism. More often, it just gets in the way of women and men living healthy, satisfying lives. While not all women experience SRFOs, they are not uncommon. Yet because of secrecy in our culture, many experiencers have been reluctant to discuss these occurrences. While most women learn to enjoy their sleep orgasms, young women, especially teen-agers, often experience distress and think that something is wrong with them.

We really do not know how common these SRFOs are in the general population because none of the large surveys with representative samples have inquired about this response. The last person to study this in-depth was Alfred Kinsey, who published his Report on Women in 1953. Based on his survey responses, he estimated that, of women who sometimes dream about sex, approximately 37% will dream to orgasm by age 45; 41% at some time in their life. Today we know that almost all women dream about sex sometime in their life, so this would mean that approximately 40% of women might experience SRFOs.   It is possible that this figure is even higher today. My survey suggests that dreams, per se, are probably not as much of a causative factor as Kinsey believed. We have learned so much more about human physiology since then.   Nonetheless, I agree with Kinsey's conclusion that there is no single causative factor, or cluster of factors, that predicts the occurrence of SRFOs in any individual's history.

In many cases, female sexuality is as much a mystery to women as it is to men. In fact, usually it has been men, like Alfred Kinsey, who have led the way in revealing women to themselves. In this book, on this topic, I am letting the women lead. Although my online survey did not require narrative comment, many women chose to offer a wide range of commentary regarding their SRFOs and dreams. The result is a level of candor that might be surprising to some readers. I hope that it is also enlightening.

I think that some of the statistics are likewise enlightening. I personally have been surprised by several trends in the data, including the very young ages at which so many respondents started experiencing SRFOs, the numbers of women who have experienced their first orgasms ever as SRFOs, and the numbers who have experienced SRFOs as their ONLY orgasms ever at any age. And while Kinsey noted that sleep orgasms seemed to peak for women in the 40 to 55 age range, the peaks today seem to be even later.

Although it is impossible to say with certainty due to lack of more comprehensive surveys, it appears that the active and accumulative incidences of these orgasms, provoked without any physical stimulation, are increasing. It is definitely time to "lift the veils."

Comments from Survey Respondents:

I'm so glad you are doing this study! I am a female who has had lucid wet dreams and always thought it was out of character because I have only heard about men having them. Also, many men do not realize that women can also experience this. I'm going to write about it in my blog. (age 21)

I think it's great that more research is being done on this topic, and I hope that more people will become aware of the existence of female sleep orgasms. (age 26)

Thank you for doing this survey. It is tremendous that you are doing this much needed research. I was appalled to google orgasm... for women and see how little research has actually been done. The information that is out there for women to read, especially young women, seems to be focused almost exclusively on male sexual experience. Women need to feel supported in their sexual experiences so that all of us can enjoy the great gift our bodies give us. Thank you once more so much! (age 31)

Thank you for doing this research! There is more to it than meets the eye. (age 31)

Up until a few years ago, I thought all women had them. I figured that if I had them, other people did. Then I was at a gathering of women and someone related a tale about a pregnant friend who was having them and all the women there reacted with amazement that this was possible. I was dumbfounded that I was the only one in a group of 6 women who had had one, and had them semi-regularly. (age 32)

I was shocked on how little I could find...on the subject. Two different physicians I consulted said they never heard of this sort of thing. I am now just a few months from graduating Registered Nursing school and I still had a difficult time finding anything worth reading...I just wanted to thank you on your paper, I do hope there will be more research on the subject. (age 35)

Whenever I talk to other people about them they've never heard or experienced them. (age 40s)

I have only begun having orgasms in my sleep and I'm 47 years old. Anyway, I couldn't find much information and your study looks like it may be very insightful. (age 47)

It's high time for awareness. I mean I feel like a tomb raider who has discovered the Book of the World's Greatest Secret !!! (age 54)

I'm glad someone is doing research on this topic. For too long, women have been denied "permission" to have any kind of sex life. When I was growing up, this subject was taboo. (age 55)

I never knew anyone had this experience as I didn't share mine with anyone until last evening in a conversation. How surprising it was to find that you are doing research on this. Thank you. (age 62)

I have not been in any kind of sexual relationship for over 20 years, but I occasionally have srfos. I have never heard anyone talk about it, and thought I couldn't possibly be the only one to experience this...so I decided to look it up online and found your article. Yay, I am not the only one! If I was I thought too bad for the other women, because they are pleasurable. (age 67)

I just found your site. It has explained a lot. Thank you. (age 68)

Chapter 2

How *Do* Women Learn About These

Sleep-Related Orgasms?

As stated in the introduction, SRFOs are neither rare nor unhealthy. There is just not much public awareness, education, or discussion about these responses. While widespread access to the internet might be changing that somewhat, the internet's impact on my survey respondents seemed to be mostly after-the-fact. Most of my survey respondents (87%) were women who experienced a sleep orgasm at some time in their lives and turned to the internet for information. Therefore, they do not represent women in general. Only nine percent of my respondents said they had never experienced a SRFO, and had never heard of such, while four percent said they had heard of SRFOs, but never experienced one.

When I asked women who experience these how they FIRST learned about sleep-related orgasms, 93% said they "experienced one." Their first SRFOs occurred at ages from under 10 to late 50s. Some mentioned that afterwards they went online to look for information...which is how they found my survey. For the other seven percent, sources of prior information also included the internet, conversations with friends or a relative, a magazine article, or a graduate school course.

These first SRFOs were often experienced as confusing, worrisome, embarrassing, or even frightening. Numerous respondents have reported thinking that there was something wrong with them, and 13% mentioned that they thought they were the "only ones" after failing to get confirmation from friends.

The good news is that, after getting over the initial surprise, 77% of experiencers report that they "enjoy them," and 50% "look forward to them." But realistically, even over time, some women "hate" them and continue to feel embarrassed. Overwhelmingly though (56%), women are also "curious about why they occur." Throughout this book I will attempt to provide some answers.

Related Survey Responses

#14. Prior to this survey, did you know that women sometimes have sleep-related orgasms? (Asked of All Survey Repsondents: n=200)

      Yes   91%   No: 9%

#14a.   If yes, how did you first learn about sleep-related orgasms?

    .5% Sex education class
  88.0% You experienced one
          (93% of   experiencers)
   3.5% A friend told you
   4.0% You read about them in a book or
         magazine
   1.0% Your mother or older relative told
         you
   3.0% Internet, graduate school

Table 1- Previous Knowledge and Learning about SRFOs

Related Survey Responses

#17g. In general, what is your subjective reaction to these sleep-related orgasms? Check all that apply (Asked of SRFO experiencers only: n= 174)

5% You feel worried about them
16% You are confused about them
10% You are embarrassed by them
56% You are curious about why they occur
2% You are afraid of them
77% You enjoy them
13% You used to feel worried, confused, embarrassed or afraid, but you no longer are
41% You find them amusing or entertaining
50% You look forward to them
19% You actively try to make yourself have them

Table 2 – Reactions to SRFOs

As I said in the introduction, I'll let women speak for themselves. I've tried to include comments from across the age span.

I don't know why they're happening and I hate them because it's embarrassing! ... I feel that

15

this is something to do with puberty and I want it to be taught in Sex Education classes so that people are aware that girls have these unprovoked orgasms! (age 15)

So I researched these random orgasms and came across this site [...] please help me. I don't know why they're happening and I hate them 'cause it's embarrassing! (age 20)

I found your survey when I was trying to figure out what was going on with me, because I quite frankly am embarrassed about it. (age 20)

I feel that the female orgasm is stigmatized and I want that to change. I was also seeking reassurance that I wasn't alone, and now I know I'm not. (age 20)

I have never met another woman that experiences these orgasms. In fact, when I bring it up to my friends, they are all shocked and laugh. It doesn't seem like many people are aware that females can experience nocturnal orgasms. I had never heard of it before I had one and I thought I was weird for having them. I was never scared that something was wrong with me because I enjoy them. They are some of the best orgasms I have ever had. (age 21)

My friends were usually surprised, and then jealous ("all the fun and none of the work"). (age 23)

I found your survey while researching SRFO online, as I have just recently started experiencing them and had no idea it existed!! I am surprised to see how common they really are! (age 24)

I'd always assumed that this happened to all women until recently when I broached the subject with some friends for the first time. They were shocked when I said it happened to me and thought I was joking. When they realized I was serious, they were intrigued and even jealous! (age 27)

I always considered these [SRFOs] to be one of my special magical powers. (age 29)

I have no personal anecdotal experience of meeting any other women who have this problem/good fortune. (age 31)

I never considered nocturnal orgasms as anything out of the ordinary. I didn't pay them much attention. (age 34)

What interesting research. I always knew that if I had them others must, but I did consider myself to be very lucky. (age 35)

I came across your page, and just wanted to say I was really impressed, and you cleared up so many questions for me...Thank you very much! (age 36)

I very much look forward to the sleeping, dreaming, lucid dreaming, and just upon waking orgasms. There is no need for touch. It's all in my head. (age 36)

I noticed recently I have been having orgasms in my sleep but I wake up feeling good and happy. This has only been occurring in the last year more frequently. I'm not complaining :) but I'm just curious as to what makes it happen. (age 36)

I had heard long ago that males did, and thought it might be possible for females as well. (age 37)

Waking up during an orgasm from a dream, or even if I do not remember the dream, has been extremely intense and wonderful. I enjoy having spontaneous orgasm and the ability to experience an orgasm without physical stimulation. (age 37)

I thought I was the only one, until a friend mentioned that she has them too. So I went online, and discovered that many other women have [them], that it's pretty common. That's when I saw your survey. (age 41)

I was so happy to run across your website. I had no idea that women can experience orgasm in their sleep. I mentioned it to my husband and a bunch of my girlfriends and everybody thinks I'm crazy and that there is no way women can have a "real" orgasm in their sleep! That's okay, I will just keep enjoying! Thanks for the information. I started experiencing SRFOs in 30s...more in 40s. (age 43)

I HATE this. I wanted to know more about it, in large part to see if there was a way to stop it. (age 51)

It is just the strangest thing because I've NEVER ONCE heard a woman speak of this...Never! Too bewildering for me to comprehend that this has never come up in my lifetime of being very out in the World! I am now 54 and still feel the same sexual urges I did in my 20's and I've already completed Menopause in my mid 40's... PS. I've now ruled out being crazy (age 54)

I began experiencing SFRO's several years ago. I am now 55 and think it began in my mid to late 40's. I'm happily married and my husband thinks SRFO's are wonderful and so do I. Any day beginning with an SFRO is a wonderful day! (age 55)

I experience orgasm on waking. I have done so for many years. I think it started when my husband became ill. I was widowed at 49 I am now 65. It happened this week. I lay back and enjoy it. It is very rare. I love it and wake very satisfied... I never told anyone, not girlfriends or grown daughters. I find it embarrassing [to talk about]. (age 65)

I am a 64 year old post menopausal woman, who experiences these from time to time (only sometimes related to dreams). In speaking with doctors, I have not received much help in understanding this phenomenon or the accompanying effects I experience. (age 64)

Other than to say that this is an unusual topic (to me), nothing else to relate except to say that the sleep orgasms were pleasant, smooth, and not long enough or frequent enough ☺. (age 65)

I went to my 50th high school reunion. I shared a hotel room with a female friend I have known since we were 11 years old. I awoke, after having a beautiful SRFO. I had the courage to ask her if she ever experienced these. She said, "Hell, yes! And, they're always better than the awake ones ever were!" Thanks for letting me know I'm normal! (age 68)

Chapter 3

What Shall We Call These?

Sleep-Related Female Orgasms (SRFOs)

One reason that it has been hard to talk about these sleep-related orgasms is that women have not been taught what to call them, since this topic is not included in sex education classes.

The most common terminology in the professional literature is "female nocturnal orgasm." This really is not accurate because these sleep-related orgasms also occur during daytime naps (and nocturnal sounds a little spooky). They are not a function of night-time or darkness.

Most of our information about these orgasms comes from Alfred Kinsey's survey of almost 6,000 Caucasian American women in the late 1940s and early 50s, published in 1953 as *Sexual Behavior in the Human Female*. There has been very little research or writing on this topic since Kinsey. Our collective knowledge base about women's health and sexuality, and our understandings in many of the fields related to sleep-related orgasms, has expanded tremendously over the past 60+ years, and it's time to update our understanding of this response also.

Kinsey used the term "nocturnal orgasm" in his narrative. His chapter title was "Nocturnal Sex Dreams," and his formal designation was "sex dreams with orgasm." However, even in Kinsey's research, dream awareness did not always precede the experience of orgasm. In my current survey, fifty percent of experiencers report times when there was no dream awareness at all preceding their orgasms.

Nonetheless, names which are sometimes used include: sleep orgasms, dream orgasms, spontaneous orgasms, unconscious orgasms, compensatory orgasms, nocturnal pollutions, or female wet dreams. For various reasons, none of these terms are totally accurate.

A 1986 study by Barbara Wells sought to define this response more rigorously for research purposes, based on the subjective experience. While she used the inaccurate designation of "female nocturnal orgasm," she defined the experience as "when sexual arousal occurs during sleep and wakes one to perceive the experience of orgasm" (Wells 1986, 425). She comments further that "Waking to, with, or from orgasm initiated during sleep seemed a necessary distinction to make for this type of survey research with women . . . [since] even employing the discovery of vaginal secretions as the indicator of nocturnal orgasm is inconclusive evidence that orgasm, or even sexual excitement, has occurred during sleep" (Wells 1986, 425).

The shift in awareness from sleep to wakefulness or awareness is an important factor in both identifying and understanding this response. Therefore, the designation "awakening orgasms" would be accurate and useful if it did not carry so many other connotations. (King 2006, 10)

We now know that these awakening orgasms occur during the REM (Rapid Eye Movement) stage of sleep which is associated with dreaming and paralysis of the voluntary muscles (so we can't act out our dreams). This research regarding sleep cycles was not available at the time Kinsey did his study.

The REM periods usually occur four or five times in a full night of sleep, and become longer toward morning. This is the stage of sleep that normally precedes morning awakening. However, since the REM periods occur several times during the night, some women will experience SRFOs several times during the same night when causal factors are present. If these occur during early parts of the night, women often become aware of having an orgasm, and then roll over and go back to sleep. The role of the sleep cycle is discussed more fully in Chapter 9.

The genitals of both men and women naturally engorge during the REM stages of sleep. This is widely recognized for men since their genitals are external, and upon awakening, men frequently have an erection. Sleep lab studies have shown that women likewise experience genital swelling and lubrication during REM, although it is not as noticeable, even to women (Fisher et al. 1983, 97). We could call these "REM-state orgasms," but few women would be likely to do a google-search for that designation. One of my respondents commented on this:

> I am currently teaching a Psychology course to juniors and seniors in high school. The textbook I am using mentions that males have erections during REM sleep and I began to wonder if females experience orgasms or arousal during REM sleep too - so I went on-line and found your web-site. My textbook does not address this.

In consultation with my Ph.D. dissertation committee chairman, Dr. Janice Epp, the designation which I introduced in my 2006 dissertation was "Sleep-Related Female Orgasms"

(SRFOs). This seems to have caught on in the blogs, so I'll stick with it as a generic reference to these awakening orgasms. Realistically, however, it is possible, though uncommon, to experience a REM-state orgasm without being aware of it. It is also possible to dream about having an orgasm without actually having a real, physical orgasm.

There are other categories of female orgasms that occur during the NREM (Non Rapid Eye Movement) stage of sleep. These are significantly different and sometimes problematic. These will be also be discussed in Chapter 9.

Meanwhile, here are some related comments from survey participants:

> Almost every time I eat cereal and take a nap...after, I have an orgasm while asleep. I have no idea why this is! (age 25)

> One of the most common times for me is during naps. (age 25)

> Until recently I remember dreaming about having orgasms, but in the past few months I have been waking up in the middle and at the end of an orgasm. I had one last night and when I wake up after having them I immediately have the urge to go back to sleep. (age 23)

> Once when I was a teenager it happened when I was having a nap on the deck while my mom and a friend were having tea not ten feet away from me. (age 30)

> Only in the last few years have I been able to have a complete orgasm during sleep. For

many years before that I would always wake up before finishing (climaxing). (age 31)

They have only ever occurred on the odd occasion when I take a nap during the day. (age 32)

I haven't been able to find much information online about this, but when I experience arousal in my dreams I almost always have multiple (consecutive) nocturnal orgasms. I have them at least once or twice a month and up to 6 or 7 orgasms in a row in my dreams. A lot of the time there is no visually stimulating sexual content in my dreams. (age 22)

I had three just this am. I can't remember a time that I haven't had them. (age 36)

I have SRFOs fairly often, I would say, at least a couple of times a month on average. But it did happen 3 times in one night, once. (age 44)

EXAMPLES of SRFOs

Due to the general lack of awareness regarding SRFOs, I'm including a few examples which show some of the varying elements and qualities which women report. They will also provide reference points for future discussion.

Example #1: The first example is from my personal experience, and took place during the months in which I was writing my dissertation. It is a classic example of an SRFO preceded by a simple, overtly sexual dream. Of the SRFO experiencers from my survey, 90% report that sometimes these SRFOs are preceded by awareness of an erotic dream. In this example, it is interesting in that both the experience and the dream content took place on bright, sunny afternoons, thus highlighting the error of "nocturnal" as a designation.

I was away from home, in the second week of a two-week business trip. I had an opportunity to take a nap following a late lunch. While sleeping, I became aware of a vivid, though not fully lucid, dream in which I was talking to a group of people on an outdoor pool deck adjacent to a large building like a hotel lobby. This felt like an informal reception or cocktail party. I was talking about my dissertation. One man in the group started talking to me. I could see him and hear him, but I could not comprehend what he was saying. So I moved closer to him and sat on a lounge chair next to him. At this point he moved on top of me and began sexual behavior. This surprised me, and I felt concerned about being in a very public place. I then felt somewhat comforted by noticing a large potted plant shielding us from view. Contact with him felt very good and my body quickly began to orgasm both in the dream and physically.

This woke me up. I noticed that I could shift my awareness back and forth between normal waking awareness and the multi-sensory dream awareness. I could not, however, move the dream forward. It stopped during orgasm, at the point at which I was awakened. I stayed in bed for a while letting my body calm down, and reflecting on the experience. I noted that this occurred approximately 1 hour and 20 minutes into sleep . . . a normal time for REM stage sleep. I also noted that I had not been aware of any sexual feelings or intention prior to the nap or during the first part of the dream. The time between contact and orgasm seemed very brief, probably less than ten seconds.

Example #2: As mentioned earlier in this chapter, 50% of the SRFO experiencers from my survey reported times when they awakened into orgasm without any preceding dream awareness at all. In Kinsey's study, only one per cent reported these cases. This might have been a result of how his question was framed, since he began his inquiry by asking about sexual dreams, and used the designation, "dreams with orgasm."

These experiences can be quite disorienting at first. Here's an example which is essentially the sound-track of my own thinking as I came into awareness during an orgasm which was not preceded by a dream.

Yikes! What's happening? Where am I? O my God! I'm exploding into a million pieces. Ahhhhhhhhhhhhhh. (Energy rushes, followed by jerk, jerk, jerk . . . dawning awareness of body) I think I have to pee. Man . . . I'm having an orgasm. . . . (contract, squeeze, contract, more energy sensations) Wow, this is intense! Oh my God!!! . . Wow! . . . . Whew! (Breathe, pant, pant, . . . giggle, giggle) . . . . That was fun!

Example #3: Often, the dreams which precede SRFOs are not overtly sexual. Thirty-six percent of the experiencers in my survey reported times "when the preceding dream...had no obvious erotic content." These next examples come from Gayle Delaney's book *Sexual Dreams* (1994), and show how the dreams which precede SRFOs do not appear to be sexual.

> I was swimming with a dolphin in clear water. All I did was feel him rub along my belly and. . . Well, you get the picture. (Delaney 1994, 25)

> I was on my childhood swing set teeter-totter. The experience became sexually arousing and ended with an outrageous nocturnal orgasm. (Delaney 1994, 26)

Here's one from my personal experience:

> In the dream, I was cleaning house, and just before the arousal and orgasm, I was dusting a bookcase. I love books. Could that have triggered it? Or did some part of my mind think that there was erotic content in one of those books? Or perhaps, could it have been the feather duster?

And from survey respondents:

> I had my first SRFO this afternoon. The dream wasn't erotic in the slightest. It was like my school was on a spring trip (I'm a senior in high school and part of the music department, and every year we take a spring trip) and had stopped to get food. (age 17)

> In my dream I was just talking on the phone, then... (age 40)

In my dream, I tried on a skirt in a dressing room and va-voom!!! My body was overwhelmed with orgasm energy. The skirt signified something for me as I rarely wore them. (age 31)

The role of dreams in SRFOs will be discussed further in Chapter Ten.

Chapter 4

Is There Something Wrong with Me?

This is probably the most common question which arises for the first-time sleep orgasm experiencer, regardless of age. Interestingly, this question has been debated (by men) throughout recorded history.

Aside from the facts and figures, one of Kinsey's greatest contributions to this topic was to clearly reject the idea that, for women, these orgasms represented some kind of pathology or neurotic condition. This had been a common attitude among medical professionals in the early 20th century. In fact, even among some prominent sexologists, dreaming to orgasm was viewed as "prima facie" evidence of neurosis. Because there might be some lingering confusion about this, I'm going to quote Kinsey's opinion:

> At various points in the literature the opinion has been expressed that nocturnal dreams in the female are an expression of some neurotic disturbance, and that "normal," well adjusted females do not dream to the point of orgasm. The very fact that nocturnal sex dreams are not as universal in the female as they are in the male seems to have contributed to the opinion that they are pathologic. There is a tendency to consider anything in human behavior that is unusual, not well known, or not well understood, as neurotic, psychopathic, immature, perverse, or an expression of some other sort of psychologic disturbance. Curiously enough, the persons who contend that sex dreams represent neurotic

disturbances in the female admit that it is impossible to believe that 80 per cent or more of the male population is to be considered neurotic simply because that percentage has nocturnal sex dreams which effect orgasm. (Kinsey et al. 1953, 195)

We women can all feel grateful for Kinsey's supportive understanding.

Today we know that orgasm is a healthful response, supplying our bodies and brains with more oxygen and surges of pleasurable and beneficial hormones and other neurotransmitters. There is some evidence suggesting that our brains/bodies use these SRFOs to restore a healthful balance or homeostasis during times of hormonal shifts, social change, unresolved sexual arousal, stress and anxiety, or high physical activity. I call this the Healthy Homeostasis theory, and discuss it in more detail in Chapter Nine. Today, some personality theorists even view SRFOs as indicators of high self-esteem, self-confidence, and creativity. I'll discuss more about these points in Chapter Nine also.

Despite the concern that there might be something wrong with them, very few of my survey respondents consulted with health professionals or spiritual advisors. (2% consulted physicians or gynecologists; 2.5% consulted mental health care providers; .5% consulted ministers or spiritual advisors.) When they did, responses ranged from surprise and total lack of awareness to re-assurance that they were normal. Fortunately, none of my respondents were told directly that there was something "wrong" with them or that they were abnormal in some way, although it might have been implied.

Based on the data from my survey, it is clear that the incidence patterns for female sleep orgasms have changed since Kinsey's time. Overall, it appears that more women are experiencing these at younger ages. I am now of the opinion that sleep-related orgasms have become a very natural step in the early sexual development process for today's young women. In addition, twenty–eight percent of the experiencers in my survey report that they experienced their very first orgasms this way, compared to approximately twelve percent in that category in Kinsey's research.

There are probably both cultural and hormonal reasons for this shift which will be discussed throughout this book. The Wells (1986) study showed that the incidence of SRFOs was influenced by cultural factors. Certainly our culture is filled with more sexual imagery and discussion now than in the 1940s and early 50s. In the United States we have also witnessed much earlier physiological development in young women since the 1950s, accompanied by earlier entry into puberty.

In Kinsey's time, twenty-two per cent of men experienced their first orgasm/ejaculations as sleep-related. So, it appears that the early incidence pattern for women now more closely resembles the developmental pattern for men.

Even though the early pattern for men and women is becoming more similar, there are very different patterns between men and women that emerge over the course of a lifetime. While Kinsey found that the peak incidences for men occurred in the teens and twenties, he found that the peak incidences for women occurred in the 40 to 55 age ranges, with variance based on marital history (never married, married, previously married). Today, while more women are experiencing these at younger ages, similar to Kinsey's male sample, many women do not begin experiencing these until their 40s and 50s, and the peaks might not be occurring until even later ages than Kinsey's sample (Table 11). Of course, patterns of marital history are also very different today than they were in the 1940s and 50s.

More participant comments:

I have never had sex or masturbated. I hadn't known what an orgasm felt like, so I just described these feelings to my doctor at about age 15 when these orgasms were beginning to happen. My doctor suggested that they were sleep-related orgasms and also asked about the content of my dreams. I told him that I couldn't remember my dreams and he said that it could be caused by an increase in hormones. (age 17)

Well, the reason I wanted to complete your survey was to find some comfort. I used to tell my best friend about how I'd be very horny and sexual after I wake from sleep and she was so narrow minded and said there is something wrong and only men have it like that. But I've always done such. (age 17)

I don't know what is wrong with me having these dreams and orgasms when I am trying to sleep. I hope they stop! (age 20)

I've mentioned them to my mother (44 years old) and she knew about sleep orgasms, but didn't say whether or not she also experiences them. (age 23)

I have even discussed sleep-related orgasms with friends and their response has been that it was demonic. Another friend said that doctors don't even understand dreams and they misguide people where some of these things are concerned. And yet another said that it was normal and gave me a link to an article on the internet to read about it. (age 26)

Wow! I always thought I was a little "strange," but after reading this, I realize that I was just NOT informed. What you describe has been happening to me since I was about 15 years old and has become VERY frequent lately (I'm 31). Thanks for posting this.

I was probably about 17 years old when I had my first sleep orgasm. I had no idea what it was and why I suddenly woke up for no reason. (age 32)

I read your article about female nocturnal orgasms and I just wanted you to know that it was very helpful to me to learn that it's physically normal to have them. However, I have to disagree with you about them being pleasurable as far as mentally. Mine somehow get linked up with my subconscious mind. I was molested from the age of 5 to 17 so almost every time I am aroused in my sleep I associate the orgasm with the people who molested me, which in turn usually ruins the rest of my day. (age 32)

I was so glad to read the introduction of your dissertation. I have experienced SRFO's and thought there must be something wrong with me, although they have been the coolest experiences I have had to date while sleeping! (age 35)

The older I get the more of dreams/and night waking orgasms I have experienced ... When I was younger I was embarrassed about having them during the night because in school we were not taught about female nocturnal emissions...only male. I definitely thought something was wrong and would be in denial of them occurring. (age 37)

Dr. King, I wanted to let you know that before finding your survey I thought my having orgasms during sleep was not normal. I felt ashamed and embarrassed. (early 40s)

I never worried or felt guilty about sleep orgasms but I did wonder what caused them and why they didn't happen more often ☺. (age 49)

Just this past month, during my pap exam, I found the courage to FINALLY ask my gyn about this phenomena. I was worried that I was "not normal", since having asked [some] very stable friends if they've ever experienced these. (One has, others have not.) He told me that they are quite normal, and that he hopes that I enjoy them. (age 54)

Thank you, Dr. Franceen for your feedback on the survey I took. I found it to be immensely helpful, and normalizing. (age 54)

My male primary care physician told me about 5 years ago that this was completely normal. I don't care if it's normal or not - I enjoy it! (age 55)

Chapter 5

How Common Are These SRFOs?

SURVEY DATA FROM KINSEY

In the 1953 report, *Sexual Behavior in the Human Female,* Alfred Kinsey and his team devoted an entire chapter to detailed statistics, analysis and commentary about "nocturnal sex dreams" and "dreams with orgasm." The most frequently cited statistic from Kinsey is that that 37% of his sample of women *who dreamed about sex,* experienced these orgasms by age 45, increasing to about 41% at any age. Understanding this statistic requires further investigation. Kinsey estimated that 70% of women, and almost 100% of men, dream about sex. Kinsey used two different populations of women for this chapter. Twenty percent of his group of 5628 Caucasian women, and 22% of his total population of 7789 women (including women prisoners and "Negroes") reported dreaming to orgasm at some time in their lives.

These figures are undoubtedly higher today due to both cultural and biological influences. For example, since the 1980s, dream studies have shown that almost ALL women, as well as men, sometimes dream about sex. Of my survey respondents, 96.5% report that they sometimes dream about sex, and of the remaining 3.5%, over half report experiencing SRFOs! However, over the years, none of the large surveys of sexual behavior which have used representative samples of women have asked about these orgasms. Therefore, we don't have data that would allow us to discover a current, accurate figure.

In fact, since Kinsey, there have been no detailed surveys regarding this topic (other than mine) which include healthy women over college age, despite the fact that Kinsey noted repeatedly that the total percentage of women in his sample experiencing these orgasms (the *accumulative incidence*) increased as women aged, at least until age 65. In other words, while some women start to experience these at ages under 10, significant numbers of women don't start to experience these until their 40s, 50s, or even older.

The level of continuing SRFO activity throughout the lifespan is one way in which this female response is very different than male "wet dreams" which are experienced by over 80% of all men in their teens and early 20s (Kinsey) and then typically decline rapidly in frequency.

MY SURVEY

Of the first 200 responses to my survey, 174 women, or 87%, reported experiencing SRFOs. Remember, these respondents do not represent women in general. My survey respondents range in age from 15 to 85, with 54% under age 40, and 46% age 40 and above. Racially or ethnically, they identified themselves as 80% Caucasian, 5% African – American, 5% Hispanic, 5% Asian ancestry, and 5% multi-racial or other. Based on their comments, it is clear to me that many of these survey respondents were experiencing SRFOs and started looking online for information. Therefore, I assume that 87% is a higher percentage of SRFO experiencers than is found in the general population.

I achieved this 87% by asking three questions about experiences with sleep orgasms: those preceded by an erotic dream; those preceded by no dream awareness; and those preceded by dreams without obvious sexual content. Some women responded "yes" to all three categories, while others responded "yes" to one or two categories. This series of questions yielded 174 individual SRFO experiencers. In the chart below, I have also included the percentage of experiencers who responded "yes" to each category.

Survey Responses (n=200)

11. Have you ever had a sexual dream that caused you to wake up having a physical orgasm?

Yes: 78%   No: 22%   (90% of experiencers)

12. Have you ever been awakened from sleep by a physical orgasm without awareness of a preceding dream?

Yes: 43.5% No: 56.5% (50% of experiencers)

13. Have you ever been awakened from sleep by a physical orgasm preceded by a dream without any obvious sexual or erotic content?

Yes: 31.5% No: 68.5% (36% of experiencers)

Table 3 – Experience of SRFOs with and without Erotic Dreams

Since late 2006, when I first posted my dissertation information and survey, I have seen two other online surveys which simply asked women if they had ever experienced a sleep orgasm. Both of these had "yes" responses of around 80%. I suspect that their respondents were also *experiencers* looking for information.

Since I am not associated with a university, I do not have access to any kind of representative sample of women who could be "required" to complete my detailed survey. All of my respondents provided information on a voluntary basis according to their interest in the topic. In some cases, when I have talked with groups of women about other topics, I have offered them the opportunity to complete my survey. A few have, and many have declined.

Another reason I think this 87% figure is too high to represent incidence in the general population is that so many women whom I meet have never even heard of sleep-related orgasms. This figure is close to 30% in my informal surveys. In my online survey, the respondents who never experienced a SRFO and did not know that such orgasms occur, equals about 9%.

Nonetheless, in Kinsey's time over 83% of men reported experiencing these by age 45, with peaks in the teens and twenties (Kinsey et al. 1953, 215). Since the incidence rates at lower ages have increased for women, it may be that at some time in the future, the overall incidence rate for women will really be over 80%.

Despite the lack of solid current research regarding accumulative incidence in the general population, there are several clues that clearly suggest a higher incidence today at younger ages than in Kinsey's time. Some of this comes from following trend lines from two studies of college age women done in 1976 (Henton) and 1986 (Wells). Some of these clues also come from the details of age and circumstance in my current survey.

AGE OF ONSET

Kinsey's data indicated that 8% of his sexual dreamers, or 6% of his total population of women, reported "dreams with orgasm" by age 20 (Kinsey et al. 1953, 216). A 1976 study by Henton surveyed 774 African American undergraduate students and revealed that 22 percent reported the experience of nocturnal orgasm by undergraduate ages. The Wells study (1986) included 245 undergraduate and graduate school women, average age: 22.14. In her study, 37 percent had experienced these orgasms by that age. Well's analysis of factors associated with this response showed that the incidence is probably influenced more by social and cultural factors than behavioral factors. However, it is likely that even education, and possibly intelligence, are factors that influence the incidence of this response (See Chapter Nine). While these three studies are not totally comparable, and none are truly representative samples, they do suggest a rapidly increasing incidence of SRFOs among *young* women over the period of 1953 to 1986, the period of the sexual revolution in American culture.

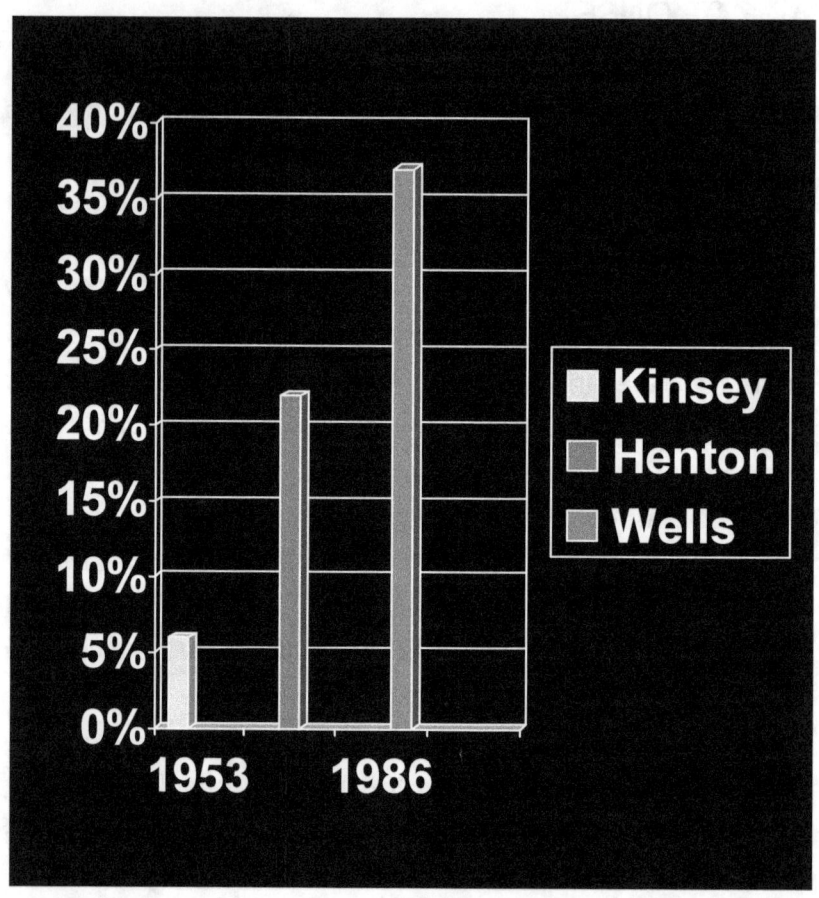

Illustration 1 – Incidence of SRFOs among young women 1953-1986

If I look at Kinsey's SRFO *experiencers* (initial Caucasian sample), I see that 19.5 % began to experience SRFOs by age 20. Many of my SRFO experiencers began experiencing them at younger ages than Kinsey's sample, with 20% experiencing them by age 15, and an additional 22% by age 20. This means that 42% of my experiencer group had SRFOs by age

20...**over twice as many by age 20 as in Kinsey's group of experiencers.**

In Kinsey's survey, 56% of his Caucasian SRFO experiencers reported nocturnal orgasms by age 30. Of my SRFO experiencers, a total of 79% experienced them by age 30.

Survey Responses (n=174)

17c. At what age do you first remember experiencing a sleep-related orgasm? (n=174)

  5% Under age 10
15% Between ages 11 and 15
22% Between ages 16 and 20
37% Between 21 and 30
12% Between 31 and 40
  7% Between 41 and 50
  1% Between 51 and 60
  0% Between 61 and 70
  1% Can't remember

Table 4 – Age of First SRFO

FIRST ORGASMS

Perhaps the most interesting comparison to Kinsey's data that I can make is the response to the question, "Did you experience your first orgasm as a result of a dream or awakening from sleep?" Kinsey found that 5% of a sample of 3826 women experienced sleep orgasms before ever experiencing a waking orgasm (Kinsey et al. 1953, 545-Table

148). Extrapolating a bit, this would mean that approximately 12% of Kinsey's Caucasian SRFO *experiencers*, experienced their first orgasm this way. As mentioned in Chapter 3, in my survey, 28% of women who reported experiencing SRFOs, experienced their FIRST orgasm this way. These occurred at ages under 10 to late 40s. **This is a very significant difference between the 1940s-50s and now.** Combined with the youthfulness of experiencers, this information screams for inclusion in sex education classes.   In Kinsey's data, 22% of young men reported experiencing their first orgasms/ejaculations as sleep-related. I have not seen any recent data for young men.

Survey Response:
Asked of SRFO experiencers only (n=174)

17e. Did you experience your first orgasm as a result of a dream or awakening from sleep?

Yes: 28%   No: 72%

Table 5 – First Orgasm Ever as SRFO

Of course, most women who experience their first orgasm as an SRFO, are easily able to begin experiencing orgasm while awake. However, this is not always the case. Ten percent of the SRFO experiencers in my survey report that these are the ONLY orgasms that they have ever experienced at any age. They have not been able to experience orgasm while awake through masturbation or with a partner. While some of these respondents are very young women who are not yet sexually active, most are in their late 20s or 30s living with partners and children. A few are over age 50. This category of respondents has been receiving a lot of attention recently in online blogs, and I will discuss this situation more thoroughly in Chapter 11.

Often, the ability to experience orgasm while awake initially begins through masturbation. A few sex researchers, including Masters and Johnson, have commented that sometimes the arousal of waking masturbation or other sexual contact, **with or without** orgasm might contribute to the experience of SRFOs.

Comments from Survey Respondents:

> Only as of recent have I begun to experience [SRFOs]... I will also note that I have never experienced sex with a partner, nor have I ever achieved orgasm through masturbation [...] I feel there may be a correlation between sleep related orgasms for me and the lack of satisfaction during self pleasure. (age 19)

> I was 11 when I discovered orgasms, but it was just a few days after I had my very first one (...awake) that I started having them in my sleep nightly. (age 19)

> I found your survey when I was trying to figure out what was going on with me, because I quite frankly am embarrassed about it. I am a virgin and ... have had no interest in sex what so ever. I want to wait 'til marriage but the whole process disgusts me! (age 20)

> I was around 5 when I had my first sleep-related orgasm (and my very first orgasm too).

I don't remember much about it, I just remember waking up to a classic orgasm, with no dream involved. This was around the time when one of my older friends had started telling me about sex. Although I do remember having sexual thoughts as early as 4 or 5. After the first orgasm, I didn't have another orgasm until I was 11. About a month after I had been practicing (and succeeding) with physical clitoral stimulation, I had my second sleep-related orgasm. I, again, don't remember the dream, but this time I knew there was a dream. (age 20)

The first time I had them was summer '08 and I was a virgin still. (age 23)

I had my first orgasm in the 6th grade while sleeping. (age 28)

I've only discussed sleep related orgasms with a few friends since they're a new thing for me, but just from that it seems to be a more rarely occurring thing than the initial survey results suggest. (age 23)

I wake up from sleep and some waves and buildup occur and then I have an orgasm. (age 28)

Chapter 6

How Do I Know if I'm Having an Orgasm?

Both Wells (1986) and Kinsey (1953) assumed that women were capable of determining for themselves whether or not orgasm had occurred. Nonetheless, as a sex therapist, one of the most common questions I receive is "How do I know if I had an orgasm?" This is commonly asked in reference to waking sexual responses, but is even more relevant to SRFOs, especially if one has never had waking sex or orgasm.

The experience of orgasm is actually highly subjective and varies tremendously for women over the course of a lifetime with different circumstances and different partners. Back in Kinsey's time, some people even doubted that women really have orgasms. And still today, there is some disagreement among sexologists about the nature of orgasm. The ground-breaking research of Masters and Johnson in the 1960s, and Shere Hite in the 1970s, clarified much about female orgasm.

Masters and Johnson (1966) described the Human Sexual Response Cycle, identifying the stages as *excitement* phase, *plateau* phase, *orgasmic* phase and *resolution* phase. They described the physiological changes associated with each phase for men and women. Helen Singer Kaplan modified this cycle based on her clinical work with women to include *desire* as the first phase, followed by *excitement* and *orgasm*. For this discussion, it is helpful to review some of the currently recognized elements of the orgasm phase.

ELEMENTS OF ORGASM

I will begin with some segments from my first book:

Since 1966, the Masters and Johnson definition has been the primary physiological standard: "The outer third of the vagina . . . contracts strongly in a regularly recurring pattern . . . The contractions have onset at 0.8-second intervals and recur within a normal range of a minimum of three to five, up to a maximum of 10-15 times with each individual orgasmic experience" (Masters and Johnson 1966, 77-78). Masters and Johnson noted numerous other physiological elements which commonly occur, including contractions of the uterus and the anal and urethral sphincters, elevated heart rate and blood pressure, vasocongestion, skin flushing, and myotonia (Masters and Johnson 1966). Other researchers have noted increased pupil diameter (Wagner 1973), elevated pain thresholds (Whipple and Komisaruk 1985, 1988), a shift in brain laterality (Cohen et al. 1976), multiple changes in neurochemistry, significant deactivation of numerous brain structures (Holstege 2005a), and a wide variety of other physiological elements including increased electrical activity within the vagina (Shafik et al. 2004).

*Helen Singer Kaplan emphasized that "the orgasm is, after all, a **reflex** [emphasis mine] and as such has a sensory and a motor component" (Kaplan 1974, 29) (from King 2006, 11).*

A *reflex* is "an involuntary and nearly instantaneous movement in response to a stimulus" (Purves 2004). Researchers are still debating the specific sensory and motor components in waking orgasms, and some researchers today disagree with the designation of orgasm as a reflex. Nonetheless, the "involuntary and nearly instantaneous movement" of orgasm is very evident in SRFOs, especially when both genital stimulation and cognitive precursors are absent. Even when cognitive precursors (awareness of dreams) exist, the speed and intensity of the orgasmic reflex is often a surprise. The stimuli which evoke this response in SRFOs apparently lie in the mind, brain, and nervous system.

One of today's outstanding sexological researchers, Cindy Meston at the University of Texas at Austin, included the following comprehensive definition of orgasm in a recent paper on female orgasmic disorder.

> Orgasm is a sensation of intense pleasure creating an altered consciousness state accompanied by pelvic striated circumvaginal musculature and uterine/anal contractions and myotonia that resolves sexually-induced vasocongestion and induces well-being/contentment. (Meston et al. 2004, 66)

For these massive physiological changes to be considered intensely pleasurable is ultimately a subjective interpretation/perception (Whipple et al. 1992, and others). A recent study suggests that for both men and women, "the subjective experience of orgasmic pleasure and satisfaction depends more on psychological and psychosocial than on physical factors" (Mah and Yitzchak 2005, 187)(from King 2006, 12).

On the other hand, many of the physiological changes, from release of physical tension to the increase in dopamine, norepinephrine, and oxytocin, contribute directly to feelings of "well-being/ contentment."

For purposes of this discussion, perhaps the most interesting part of the Meston et al. definition is the reference

51

to orgasm as "creating an altered consciousness state" (Meston et al. 2004, 66). In the case of SRFOs, consciousness alters from sleep to wakefulness. Awareness often shifts from the bizarreness of a dream scenario to normal reality. Given that "dreaming is considered to be an altered state of consciousness . . . [and] lucid dreams can be considered an altered state of dreaming" (Van de Castle 1994, 444), there are multiple consciousness altering factors at play in the SRFO...

There is one other element of orgasm that merits attention in the exploration of SRFOs [. . .] The notion of sexual energy has lost favor in sexological research because, to date, there is no way to observe or quantify this energy. Nonetheless, the experience of energy movement, whether described as sexual energy or simply life energy, is well known to many, in both waking sex and SRFOs. The yogic traditions of the East acknowledge this energy movement in Tantric sex practices. As interpreted by sex therapist Judy Kuriansky, "Tantric sex redefines what sex is – not as an action, but as movement of energy within you individually, and between you and your partner. The practices guide you to generate sexual energy, transform it into love energy, and transmit it to your partner and even to the universe" (Kuriansky 2002, 24)(from King 2006, 13-15).

THE EXPERIENCE OF ORGASM

Despite the many common elements of orgasm, as mentioned earlier, not all orgasms are experienced in the same way. Although, our subjective experiences of orgasm might vary widely, it does appear that orgasm typically becomes easier for women over the lifespan as a result of familiarity and learning. In discussing the *physiological* propensity toward orgasm within a single sexual experience, Dr. Mary Ann Sherfey noted that, "The more orgasms a woman has, the stronger they become; the more orgasms she has, the more she *can* have" (Sherfey 1972, 112).

This idea really applies not only to an individual love-making session, but to the journey over time. Not surprisingly, the most recent National Survey of Sexual Health and Behavior (NSSHB) showed that the oldest category of women studied (ages 50-59) had the highest rate of orgasm in their most recent partnered sex experience: 70.7% vs. 57.8% in the age 25-29 category (Herbenick et al. 2010, 353). When physiological familiarity is combined with one's expanding knowledge, imagination, and creativity, many possibilities emerge. For example, many people today find new, powerful, and satisfying variations in Tantric and Sacred Sex practices. Others create richer, more varied mental fantasies. Others feel more confident experimenting with new sexual behaviors.

Orgasms are experienced in so many different ways. As educator Rebecca Chalker notes in her excellent book, *The Clitoral Truth*:

> There are many different types: mini-orgasms; maxi-orgasms; quickie orgasms; explosive orgasms; multiple orgasms, dry, non-ejaculatory orgasms; extended orgasms, which can last anywhere from a few minutes to several hours; focused orgasm (experienced primarily in the genitals); irradiating orgasms, which may be felt in the pelvis and upper thighs; full-body orgasms; out-of-body orgasm (feels like it, anyway); well-earned orgasms; unconscious orgasms (the fabled "wet dreams," which may or may not involve genital

53

engorgement and occur in both women and men); even involuntary orgasms, and so on...only you can be the judge of the quality of an orgasm. In my view, there are not "bad' orgasms, just shorter, longer, weaker, stronger, and when time and circumstances permit, the much vaunted Vesuvian ones (Chalker 2000, 58).

Ninety-nine per cent of my first 200 survey respondents reported that they have experienced orgasm, either while awake or through sleep. This is not typical of the general population. With a representative sample of women, usually between eight to fifteen percent report that they have never experienced orgasm. (A few writers suggest that this figure might even be much higher.)

If you recall from the previous chapter, ten percent of the SRFO experiencers in my survey report that orgasms initiated in sleep are the ONLY orgasms that they have EVER experienced. They comprise most of the 9% "No" response in the chart below.

Related Survey Responses (n=200)

15. Are you able to experience sexual orgasms when you are awake? Yes: 91%   No: 9%

15a. If yes, please indicate all the ways in which you are able to experience orgasm.

74% Through masturbation
75% Through fantasy & masturbation combined
65% Through manual stimulation by a partner
60% Through oral stimulation by a partner
48% Through vaginal stimulation by partner

Table 6 – Waking Orgasmic Response by Behaviors

16. At what age did you experience your first orgasm?

21% Under age 10
32% Between ages 11 and 15
27% Between ages 16 and 20
19% Between ages 21 and 30
0% Between ages 31 and 40
1% Between 41 and 50

Table 7 – Age of First Orgasm

Chapter 7

Why Are My Sleep Orgasms So Intense?

Many women report that sleep-related orgasms are experienced as stronger or more intense...especially the speed of arousal and strength of the contractions. There are several possible reasons for this, and I will offer a few thoughts for consideration. At this point, though, I will be entering into more speculative territory, because a thorough discussion requires more knowledge of neuro-physiology and the research simply has not been done.

LACK OF INHIBITIONS AND VOLUNTARY MUSCLE CONTROL

A primary reason for increased intensity is probably the lack of voluntary muscle control that accompanies REM sleep, combined with the frequent lack of conscious, psychological inhibition in a non-lucid dream. Kinsey did not have access to our current physiological understandings about REM sleep; however, he commented based on the psychological factors:

> Sexual responses in sleep may differ, however, from the responses which one makes when awake, in the fact that the learned controls and inhibitions which an individual has acquired in the course of his or her lifetime are less likely to operate in sleep. The content of the dream, the speed of the response, and the abandon of the activity in orgasm may be less obstructed by rational controls . . . One of the most characteristic aspects of nocturnal sex dreams is

the speed with which they carry the individual to orgasm, even though he or she may be quite slow in response while awake. An occasional female who finds it difficult to release her inhibitions and reach orgasm while awake may be able to reach it in sleep." (Kinsey et al. 1953, 193)

We now know from PET scans of women's brains during waking orgasm that a release of conscious control seems to be necessary to allow the reflex of orgasm to occur. The prefrontal cortex, associated with reason and behavioral control, virtually shuts down during orgasm (Holstege et al. 2005). In general, brain activity during REM often more closely resembles brain states during orgasm than ordinary wakefulness. The lack of voluntary muscle control allows the orgasm reflex to express fully without intentional moderation.

I think another reason for the experience of intensity comes from the fact that normally in sleep we do not have anything inside our vaginas. Since there is nothing for the muscles to contract against, the contractions often feel much *deeper* and stronger, as they begin in sleep, and can sometimes result in lingering muscle cramping. In many cases, it is the intensity of the contractions that shifts one into wakefulness, or at least awareness of the physical body. Even Kinsey noted that "the female is often awakened by the muscular spasms or convulsions which follow her orgasms" (Kinsey et al. 1953, 192). These deep pelvic contractions, which typically include the vagina, the uterus, and the anal and urethral sphincters, also led some of my survey respondents to comment that they had their first "vaginal" orgasms this way...or their first "full body" orgasms.

The distinction between "vaginal" and "clitoral" orgasms was first made by Sigmund Freud in 1905, and has been highly criticized by women ever since. His distinction was based on the part of the woman's body that is stimulated in order to reach orgasm. He felt that orgasm through clitoral stimulation was an immature response compared to orgasm reached through vaginal stimulation. In SRFOs, neither the clitoris nor the vagina are physically stimulated, so this distinction really does not apply. But as noted above, women tend to categorize orgasms according to how and where they *feel* them.

NERVE PATHWAYS

Another reason for the intensity of sleep orgasms is that it is likely that different nerve pathways are more involved in SRFOs than in waking orgasms. Increasingly scientists are recognizing that there is no single nerve pathway that is responsible for orgasm, and consequently no single part of the body that is solely responsible for stimulating orgasm. For example, some women have orgasmic responses to nipple stimulation. Nipples and breasts connect to the spinal column through the **intercoastal nerve**. Counting the intercoastal nerve, at this time it is thought that there are at least five major nerve pathways which play a role in female orgasm at least some of the time. This is probably what accounts for the wide variations in the experience of orgasm, as well as variety in personal erogenous zones.

Clinical sexologists recognize the clitoris as the organ of sexual pleasure for women, but most women do not realize that most of the clitoris is actually under the skin, shaped somewhat like a wishbone which runs under the outer labia and wraps around the vaginal opening toward the anus. In addition to the external clitoral glans (the "love button") and clitoral shaft and hood, it includes the engorging bulbs underneath the outer labia (lips), and also extends inward above and around the urethra. Some writers include the paraurethral glands, also known as the "female prostate" as part of the clitoris, and some writers are now referring to the *clitoral complex.* Awareness of some of these hidden clitoral structures is sometimes more predominant in SRFOs, even though there is no physical stimulation. Often, however, awareness of the vagina, uterus, and entire pelvic region is more predominant in SRFOs.

The clitoris connects to the **pudental nerve** which also has connections to the vulva, urethra, anus, and outer vagina areas. Most of the nerve endings which are stimulated by *touch* to these areas during sex or masturbation connect to the pudental nerve.

The **pelvic nerve** connects to the inner vagina, the bladder, rectum, cervix, urethra, and paraurethral glands. The **vagus nerve** connects to the uterus and cervix, as does the **hypogastric nerve**, which also connects to the paraurethral glands. In waking sex, these nerves are often stimulated by *pressure* in the vagina (or even on the abdomen) during sex, rather than the sensation of touch.

The pudental, pelvic and hypogastric nerves interact with each other in the lower part of the spinal column: S2, S3, S4 (the sacral plexus). The vagus nerve goes directly to the brain stem and by-passes the spinal column. It has been shown that many women with spinal cord injuries and paralysis are able to experience orgasm (Sipski-Alexander 2001), including orgasm in sleep (Komisaruk et al. 2010. 54). It is thought that this is due to the activity of the vagus nerve network since it does not require spinal cord mediation. Interestingly, women who can experience orgasm simply by thought or fantasy also show increased activity in the brain centers associated with the vagus nerve (Komisurak et al. 2004). This would suggest that the vagus nerve might play an important role in SRFOs, especially when there is awareness of a dream. However, 50% of the SRFO experiencers in my survey reported that sometimes they experience SRFOs without awareness of a preceding dream. Kinsey assumed that those who reported orgasms without a preceding dream simply did not remember the dream. Perhaps this is the case, although, as we will see in Chapter Nine, there are many possible factors related to these orgasmic responses besides dreams.

Three of these nerve pathways (pelvic, vagus, and hypogastric) are part of the autonomic system and not under voluntary control. Since the voluntary muscles are paralyzed during REM sleep, it is likely that SRFOs are mediated more through these nerve pathways than the pudental nerve which is part of the somatic nervous system. Our scientists are just beginning to sort out these potential orgasmic pathways, but this might be one reason why SRFOs are experienced as more intense and often described as more "vaginal." This has not actually been studied in a laboratory setting. In fact, I could only find one case ever of a woman experiencing an SRFO in a sleep lab setting (LaBerge 1983), and that was in a study of lucid dreaming.

MAPPING THE VAGINA

It seems that many writers in recent years have been mapping pressure points in the vagina. This might be due to the fact that sexologists have put so much emphasis on the clitoris over the past 30+ years, that some women (and men) feel that the vagina has been neglected. Obviously, clitoral stimulation is extremely important in waking sex and cannot be ignored. But many women also love vaginal penetration for both physical and emotional reasons. So today, there is more talk about "blended" orgasms, recognizing that there are so many possibilites as mentioned in the previous chapter. While none of these areas are physically stimulated to evoke SRFOs, one might become very much aware of them. So, I will take a moment to summarize some favorite discoveries.

Pressure against the front wall of the vagina, just an inch or two beyond the vaginal opening, can stimulate an area now called the G-spot. This is not an anatomical structure per se, but rather an area that becomes pleasurably sensitive to pressure during arousal for some women. This area has a somewhat textured surface during arousal and can easily be felt with fingers. Most of the vaginal interior is smooth. The A-spot (Anterior Fornix) is a little further inside the vagina, also on the front wall, before the cervix (the opening to the uterus). Some writers report intense arousal due to pressure in this area. During arousal, the cervix and uterus lift up, opening the vaginal pathway. The part of the cervix that protrudes into the vagina is shaped somewhat like a very small donut with a hole in the middle and has a harder surface than the surrounding vaginal walls. Many women find pressure against the outer edge of the lifted cervix, which usually occurs naturally in penis-vagina intercourse, to be pleasurable. If the cervix and vagina have not lifted, bumping against the side edge of the cervix is usually experienced as painful because it causes the entire uterus to move in an often uncomfortable manner.

The portion of the vagina beyond the cervix, which balloons or "tents" during arousal, is sometimes called the cul-de-sac (Keesling 1997). Pressure on the front wall beyond the cervix in an area called the posterior fornix, stimulates another potentially pleasurable sensation. Pressure on the **back** side of this cul-de-sac stimulates a nerve plexus which is responsible for generating waves of increased electrical activity in the vagina (Shafik et al. 2004, 2007) due to the presence of Interstitial Cells of Cajal (ICCs) in the smooth muscle cells. These cells in other parts of the body typically generate an electrical wave pattern and muscle contractions. Therefore, this area might be "responsible for the vaginal contractile activity" (Shafik et al. 2004). Barbara Keesling reported that pressure in this "cul-de-sac" can literally create the visual perception of fireworks even with one's eyes closed.. This is known as a "phosphenic" response. Perhaps we can call this upper back part of the vagina the V-Spot for voltage, vagina, or va-voom!

ORGASM THROUGH FANTASY ALONE

In my survey, 39% of respondents reported that they are sometimes able to experience orgasm as a result of waking sexual fantasy alone without any physical stimulation. This contrasts with 2% of Kinsey's sample of women. So far, I have not found any statistics on how common this ability is today in the general population. In recent years, Barry Komisaruk and Beverly Whipple have been studying brain activity associated with "thinking off." Their book, *The Orgasm Answer Guide* (2010), addresses many questions about orgasm in general.

I will address the topic of fantasy in several other parts of this book. While some fantasies might involve imagining unusual scenarios with other people, the most common form is simply *remembering* pleasurable sensations.

```
Survey Responses (n=200)

21. Have you ever experienced orgasm as a
result of waking sexual fantasy only (without
any physical stimulation)?
          Yes: 39%          No: 61%

If yes, how often?:

    22.5% Less than 10 times in life
     7.0% Usually about 1 to 5 times each year
     4.5% Usually about 6 to 12 time each year
     4.5% More than once a month
      .5% More than once a week
```

Table 8 – Ability to Experience Orgasm by Waking Fantasy Alone

Aside from the intensity of the contractions, in some cases, the intense *arousal* sensations attract the attention of SRFO experiencers and lead them into into wakefulness before the contractions begin.   And for others, it is the altered consciousness of the dream state which attracts attention and allows new kinds of perceptions and awarenesses to emerge. Overall, we women tend to classify orgasms according to how we feel or experience them, as noted above, and the combinations of our physiology and consciousness make the potential possibilities almost limitless!

Although my survey did not specifically ask about "speed," "intensity," or "energy movement," many respondents chose to comment on these qualities:

> The ones in my dreams are much more intense than any other orgasm I have been able to acquire. My partner has come very close but even his efforts can hardly compare to my dreams. (age 19)

> When they do happen, its definitely orgasmic, but (I don't really know how to put it!) they are always very much about the build up and then happen very quickly (age 20)

> The orgasm seems to come on more quickly than my waking orgasms and be more intense as well. (age 22)

> From reading people's threads on the internet, it also seems like a lot of women suggest their sleep orgasms are somehow 'stronger' or more intense than most orgasms they experience when they're awake... I would agree that the sleep related orgasms are more consistently very intense. (age 23)

> The only thing I would like to add is when these sleep-related orgasms occur, they are immediately followed by severe abdominal cramping (very painful). (age 24)

> Although I enjoy my nocturnal orgasms, I find them at times painful and intense. (age 27)

The orgasm is completely different – it feels internal and I guess this is what a vaginal orgasm feels like (I have only had a vaginal orgasm twice in my life this far). I usually have clitoral orgasms. The orgasm is much more of a whole body experience and I think, better than a clitoral orgasm. (age 28)

One thing I find interesting is that the SRFOs that I have are by far the most intense orgasms I experience in my life, in terms of sensation and physical intensity of response. (age 32)

The orgasms are through vaginal penetration in my dreams which is something I can't achieve when I'm awake. (age 34)

The orgasms are great and the last one I had two nights ago was so intense that I almost wished it would stop! After the orgasm that seemed to last forever, I then experienced "hiccup" orgasms...they just kept coming like a hiccup. I was rudely awakened by my alarm at that point. Horrific!!!! (age 36)

Waking up during an orgasm from a dream, or even if I do not remember the dream, has been extremely intense and wonderful. I enjoy having spontaneous orgasm and the ability to experience an orgasm without physical stimulation. The resulting feeling is far different from being with my partner, though intense they are not quite as fulfilling as when I am with him. (age 37)

I started experiencing sleep-related orgasms in my 30s and they seem to have intensified the last few years. I have no idea why and they're like nothing I have ever experienced. (age 39)

Exactly 4 times I have experienced very strong orgasms when I was sleeping. The feeling and the strength of pleasure was UNBEARABLE, I could not resist it and I forced myself to wake up! (mostly I am aware of the fact that I'm in my dreams) but I cannot explain how my body can experience physical sensation without physical contact! And what surprises me is that I never got wet during these orgasms, the sensation was 10 times stronger than real orgasms. I would like to know how a body can feel such physically without physical contact or is it brain that creates this sensation??? (age 42)

The surprising thing about sleep orgasms is that without any physical stimulation they can often be far more intense than orgasm by masturbation. I would say that the most intense orgasms I have experienced have been with a partner and sleep orgasms rank second. (age 48)

I am dead asleep until I realize at a more awakening point that I am actually going through an Orgasm. My vagina feels hot and contracted, and I practically wake-up due to the intensity. Then realizing that neither my husband is rubbing me or even me rubbing me. I actually move my pelvis like I'm being pumped until I finish the Orgasm. (age 55)

The orgasms are so intense that you immediately think that someone else has to be included in the moment. But in my experiences, when I am more than half asleep, and it just feels so good..... I don't fight it! I WANT TO FINISH! (age 55)

Chapter 8

Is It Possible for Women to Experience Sleep Orgasm Emissions – or "Wet" Dreams?

Fluid emissions cannot be used as an indicator of orgasm for women during wakefulness or sleep. Some women lubricate very little during arousal or orgasm. Lubrication often decreases with age, especially after menopause.

On the other hand, sometimes women produce a significant volume of fluid emissions during waking sex. While preparing my dissertation, I talked with several women who reported large fluid expulsions during SRFOs, as well. This was very surprising to them, and the fluid did not seem to be urine.

Significant fluid emissions during SRFOs have also been reported by survey respondents and others (including partners) who have emailed me with questions and comments. So, obviously, fluid emissions of varying amounts *can* occur during SRFOs.

Over the past fifteen years or so, there has been much discussion about female ejaculation, and a proliferation of books and training programs designed to teach women to "ejaculate." While there is still debate about the precise mechanisms, it has been shown that some women do expel urine from the urethra during sexual activities and orgasm, while others expel a fluid from the urethra which has a different chemical composition than urine. This other fluid contains more glucose and an enzyme called prostatic acid phosphatase (Komisaruk et al. 2010, 21). It is now thought that this fluid is produced by the paraurethral glands, sometimes called the "female prostate." Prior to this ejaculation, women often report a feeling of having to urinate.

Other women report that they sometimes "gush" a significant volume of fluid from their vaginas. There is some disagreement about the source of this fluid. Some writers think this comes through the cervix from the uterus, or is created by the cervix, and is different than the normal vaginal transdermal lubrication sometimes called "vaginal sweating" which comes through the vaginal walls. Some writers think this comes from the Skene's glands near the urethra. We know that during the time of the month around ovulation, women secrete a thicker, white, more mucus discharge from the cervix. While most of us women are used to some kind of "gushing," whether it's menstrual fluids, pre-birth amniotic water breaking, or fluids associated with sexual experiences, sometimes it is difficult to say just where it is coming from.

A variety of these responses can occur during SRFOs. In addition, it appears that women who learn to ejaculate when awake, increase their likelihood of ejaculating during SRFOs.

> Although I have become aroused a few times in my sleep it was only once I woke up to a full orgasm. This happened last year when I was 19 and was the best orgasm I've had in my life, lasting for several minutes. It seemed to have a very different quality to it than any other orgasm I have experienced. I had tears of joy

streaming down my face (something I have only experienced one other time during an orgasm). All I felt was the purest joy and ecstasy. I must have also been wetter than I have ever been as my thighs and sheets were also wet. (age 20)

For the last 6 months of my new relationship, I ejaculate almost every time my lover and I engage in sexual intercourse and we do this roughly 4 times a week. Last night I went to bed and had a thought of my lover and I having sex. I don't remember falling asleep, but I do remember waking up and catching my breath as if I were actively having sex. As I woke up, I realized I was in a pool of liquid but, I also knew it wasn't urine. As you may know, the liquid from female ejaculation has a different texture than that of urine. I was in utter shock because I just could not understand HOW I managed to ejaculate in my sleep! This experience is what brought me to your website. (age 26)

Sometimes I sleep with dreams about some porn. The next day I woke up and I found my underpants were wet. I don't know whether it is emission or not. I very much want to know what happened to myself. (age 27)

I am 40 now, and began experiencing female ejaculation about 2 years ago. Last night, after a particularly wild lovemaking session, I went to the bathroom, did my business, brushed my teeth and went to bed as usual. About 5 hours later, I woke up soaked (indicative of a nocturnal emission); I have no recollection of any dreams, and there was no odor or discoloration that would indicate urination. Is this even possible for women? I welcome the female ejaculation as a new and amazing part of my sex life, but not so sure about the involuntary aspect of dealing with them in my sleep (especially if I haven't the benefit of consciousness and joy out of the deal!)

I have always had, even in my first experiences with masturbation, easily achieved orgasms accompanied by explosive emissions. I've never had a problem with anything... until last night. I awoke to soaked pajama pants and a huge puddle on my mattress. I know the difference between urine and emissions, and was not confused at all... Yesterday was one of those frustration-in-masturbation days. (age 40)

Fluid emissions can be a source of concern to women who experience them. One woman told me that she was almost convinced that she had been inseminated in her sleep until convincing herself that the fluids did not feel, taste, or smell like semen. Sometimes partners are even more concerned. I was once asked to be an "expert" witness in a legal case involving female "nocturnal emissions." On the other hand, I had one husband rather proudly tell me that he had successfully video recorded his wife's sleep orgasm emissions.

Interestingly, Sigmund Freud thought that SRFOs might be caused by bladder fullness (Bass 1994, 491). Since SRFOs often occur toward morning, bladder fullness is frequently a co-existing condition. Freud thought that bladder fullness might be putting pressure against sensitive nerves. Some of my survey respondents chose to comment on this, and some also identified intestinal fullness or the pressures of pregnancy as possible contributors. In the next chapter I will discuss many other theories about possible causes.

> I was awake enough when the orgasm happened to first think "oh crap" and assume that what I was feeling was that I had to pee and that I was about to wet myself. I don't think I was awake enough to actually move to get up, because I didn't, and I waited a second to see if that feeling was actually a full bladder, only to realize that that was a different kind of pressure that I was feeling, and then I had a small orgasm. (age 17)

> NONE of my orgasms are physically stimulated. I wake up once a week or less, not remembering my dream, but with an orgasm. I also have the urge to urinate about a minute after waking up. (age 17)

> Sometimes I will wake up while it is happening, especially when the onset of cramping is very painful. Then I will have to urinate. Other times I will know it is happening, and immediately go back to sleep. (age 24)

> I seem to experience SRFO's more often when I have a moderate to strong urge to urinate. Didn't know if that would be helpful for you to know. I also enjoy sex more when I have at least a moderate urge to urinate. (age 26)

Chapter 9

What Causes SRFOs?

There is no single answer to this question. It is clear now that there are many factors, and combinations of factors, which influence this response. In my opinion, this is one of the main reasons that these SRFOs have not been studied. The possible causes span so many different fields of inquiry and research.

In this chapter I will review some of the theories from the past and present, look at some of the possible causal factors, including those that have been researched and those that have not, and also share some opinions from survey respondents. Consequently, this will be a long chapter! I am going to begin with a segment from the Abstract of my dissertation which provides a good overview:

The study summarizes what is known about SRFOs based on existing research and historical opinion in fields of sexology, physiology, psychology, sleep, dreaming, anthropology and spirituality. While Kinsey noted that there is no single factor or cluster of factors that is predictive of SRFOs in an individual history, the strongest predictors in his research were frequent waking orgasm and "erotic responsiveness," low availability of other psycho-sexual outlets, masturbation, and fantasy during masturbation (Kinsey et al. 1953, 212-15). Today research suggests that overall, sleep mentations are more continuous than compensatory, and that sexual content and orgasmic experience during sleep are more likely among women who think about sex when awake. Waking cognitions include memory, fantasy, desire, imagination, prosexual attitudes, knowledge of SRFOs, and familiarity/safety with sexual pleasure and the orgasmic reflex. It is likely that formal education, intelligence, personality characteristics, and other cultural factors also influence these sleep mentations. Orgasmic responses during sleep seem more likely when there is some level of autonomic nervous system arousal before sleep, including both psychological and physiological elements. Physiological elements include lingering arousal from waking orgasms or other sexual behavior; however, this arousal may also be due to hormonal fluctuations, physical exercise, or emotional states such as anxiety, or anger. In these latter cases, SRFOs might serve a compensatory role in maintaining system homeostasis. It is likely that SRFOs occur more frequently among lucid dreamers due to possible neurological conditions unique to the lucid dream state, and the conscious freedom to exercise volition by choosing pleasure. SRFOs appear to be neither unhealthy nor rare.

Today, I agree with everything I wrote then; however, my understanding of some of these points has changed, especially the last point about lucid dreaming. While some of my survey respondents indicated that they frequently enjoy SRFOs initiated in lucid dreams, some survey respondents indicated that, in many cases, lucid dreaming actually inhibits SRFOs. One reason is that, in lucid dreams, with both awareness and some degree of control or volition, the same conscious inhibitions that occur in waking life often surface. Kinsey thought that dreams, in general, were the primary cause of SRFOs. This might not be true based on newer understandings; however, dreams are sometimes an

76

important element in SRFOs, so I will give dreaming more attention in the next chapter.

OLD THEORIES
Demons

This is probably the oldest theory of all. As strange as this idea might seem to many in 2012, I feel compelled to include this since it still shows up in some current religious teachings, internet blogs, and survey respondent concerns. The notion that non-corporeal demons cause SRFOs, or the idea that there exist spiritual beings capable of having sex with humans, is as old as human history, with literary references as far back as the first written stories from the ancient Sumerian culture.

In many ancient religious traditions throughout the planet, the spiritual beings mated with humans, and their off-spring became demi-gods or political leaders. But this was not always the case.

One of the primary stories to influence Western historical beliefs about SRFOs and nocturnal emissions probably originated in the myths regarding a character named Lilith. The Jewish *Talmud,* a collection of literature from around 500 B.C to A.D 300, contains references to evil spirits and demons, and specifically mentions Lilith as the instigator of erotic dreams. She was also mentioned in the *Dead Sea Scrolls* and the Jewish *Midrash* or folktale tradition.

Re-written anonymously in the eighth to tenth century AD, as the *Alphabet of Ben Sira*, the story describes Lilith as Adam's first wife, created at the same time and in the same manner as he. The short version of the story is that she left him because he never let her be on top during sex, and went to a place where she lived with spirit beings, since she was half spirit. However, she needed semen to produce offspring. So she, and her female offspring eventually called succubi, would steal men's semen at night by having sex with them. Her male offspring, the incubi, would similarly cavort with, and occasionally impregnate, human women. Eventually, she became known as the Queen of the Demons, the mother of the Incubi and Succubi. She was also accused of killing newborns who died of the condition we today call Sudden Infant Death Syndrome. Although this story was considered "folklore," it resulted in numerous Jewish religious rituals.

In the early days of the Catholic Church, opinions regarding sexual experiences in sleep were mixed. Thanks mostly to St. Augustine, in the fifth century, the nocturnal emissions of men were viewed simply as *happenings* without any moral judgment, unless one had somehow invited or tried to cause them (Flanagan 2000, 18). But by the thirteenth century, when the Catholic Church began it's crackdown on heretics, the "demons," which had originally been viewed more as bothersome thoughts, became virtually synonymous with "the devil." During this time, even dreaming at all became evidence of heresy (Van de Castle 1994, 84). The *Malleus Maleficarum* (or *Witches' Hammer*), the written directive which began the 700 year Inquisition, included numerous passages about the innate evilness of women due to their inability to control their sexual impulses and consequently "for the sake of fulfilling their lusts they consort even with devils" (Kramer and Sprenger 1971[1486], 47). Sexual responses during sleep were considered evidence of having had sex with the devil. During these years, hundreds of thousands of people, overwhelmingly women, were tortured and put to death for this and other reasons.

In my first book I devoted a very lengthy, detailed chapter to the history of how SRFOs have been viewed from moral and spiritual perspectives in various cultures over time. As you can tell, these sleep experiences received much more public attention than they do today, but that attention was highly superstitious, fear-based, and even life-threatening. This is undoubtedly one reason why some are afraid to discuss this topic today.

Before leaving this topic, I want to mention that there is a fairly common sleep disorder called "sleep paralysis" which probably contributed to the idea of "demons." This is discussed below under the topic 'Brain Activity During Sleep."

> I am going into ministry and I am desperately seeking righteousness in all areas of my life, by God's grace. I have been having dreams lately that I know are related to the giving up of masturbation … So, waking up to an orgasm, made me first think of an Incubus, even though I don't much believe in that sort of thing. Lol. (age 19)

> I have discussed sleep-related orgasms with friends and their response has been that it was demonic. (age 26)

> I used to think that some ghost was having sex with me. And I used to be scared of them. I kicked that thought and now I look forward to them. Unfortunately it only happen 2/3/4/ time a year. I wish I could will it to happen! (age 28)

But I have to say before I do go back to sleep I have to pull my conscious self together by ruling out that there's not someone else in the room and that it's not from watching too many Ghost stories. (age 55)

When I lived in Turkey, I learned from friends that if a SRFO occurred to a Turkish woman, she blamed it on evil "cins" (pronounced "gins" and related to the word "genies.") They considered it a bad thing, and were ashamed, like they had done something wrong. So sad!! (age 68)

Pathology

Eventually, in the late eighteenth and nineteenth centuries, science, medicine, and politics came to the rescue. Sleep-related orgasms and nocturnal emissions became more of a medical concern...a physical and/or psychological pathology. This assessment gradually began to drop away for men in the early twentieth century. But as noted in Chapter Four, in 1953 Kinsey had to dispute the pathology issue regarding SRFOs for women. Nonetheless, a few medical doctors persisted with this line of thinking beyond the 1950s.

Biological Compensation

Moving further into the 20th century, the dominant theory about the cause of sleep-related orgasms and nocturnal emissions was the idea of biological compensation. Essentially, this meant that if people were abstaining from sex, or not having adequate sexual expression while awake, their bodies would compensate by sexual outlet in sleep.

This theory was very popular when Kinsey began his research. According to Kinsey's initial understanding, "the frequencies of the dreams are supposed to have an inverse relation to the frequencies of other sexual activities, thus providing a safety valve for the 'sexual energy' which accumulates when other outlets are unavailable or are not being utilized" (Kinsey et al. 1953, 207). However, Kinsey's results with women (and men) did not strongly support the compensation theory, either in frequency or circumstance, despite the fact that he included an extra 700 women prisoners in his study of "dreams with orgasm." Only 14% of his cases showed any suggestion of biological compensation, and the rates of frequency were not nearly adequate to compensate for loss of other sexual outlets.

Several researchers before Kinsey addressed this topic. Regarding women specifically, Hammer asserted "that the female who is deprived of other sexual outlets will find relief in nocturnal orgasms once every third day. Mantegazza, however, says once in four or five days." (reported in Kinsey et al. 1953, 208). These writers did not present data to support their statements, and Kinsey's frequency data was much lower than these estimates (King 2006, 27).

FREQUENCY

The frequency of SRFOs among Kinsey's sample varied among individuals, and fluctuated significantly over any individual's lifetime. Overall, "the average frequencies for those who were having [orgasmic] dreams . . . remained around 3 to 4 times per year from adolescence to the oldest age groups . . . at least to age sixty-five"(Kinsey et al. 1953, 201).   Twenty-five percent of his group reported sleep orgasms only 1 to 6 times in their entire lives (Kinsey 1953.

668). The frequencies of SRFOs among my survey respondents were more in line with the Kinsey and Wells responses; however, there was considerable variability over the lifespan associated with factors discussed later in this chapter. And of course, the very young experiencers were more likely to select the "Less than 10 times in life" category.

Survey Responses:
Asked of SRFO Experiencers Only (n=174)

17a. Have you experienced a sleep-related orgasm during the past five years?
      Yes: 95%   No: 5%

17b. With or without an accompanying dream, how often have you experienced sleep-related orgasms?

  32% Less than 10 times in life
  29% Usually about 1 to 5 times each year
  18% Usually about 6 to 12 times each
        year
  17% More than once a month
   2% More than once a week
   2% Varies too much to answer

Table 9 – Active Incidence and Frequency of SRFOs

Since biologic compensation was not the main cause of SRFOs in Kinsey's sample, what was? He found a slight positive correlation between the occurrence of masturbation, and the occurrence of fantasies in masturbation with nocturnal orgasms (Kinsey et al. 1953, 211). In addition, some of his respondents with the highest frequencies of

SRFOs were women who experienced the highest frequencies of waking orgasms. Kinsey concluded that *psychological* factors played a more significant role in SRFOs than biological compensation. He essentially felt that the dreams themselves were the cause of the SRFOs, even when women did not remember the dreams. Further, he thought that these dreams depended largely on psychological factors including imagination and memory (based on sexual experience including masturbation and marital history). However, he also noted that both physiological and psychological factors could operate in different ways at different times for even the same subjects. (Kinsey et al. 1953, 212).

In my current survey, a few of the comments suggested biological compensation. More commonly, *emotional* or *psychological compensation* showed up in more pronounced ways, especially between or following the end of relationships. When I asked respondents to indicate the kinds of conditions when SRFOs have been most common for them, 38.5% included times "when between, or without, a sexual relationship." My respondents could select as many conditions as they desired, so this figure does not represent a percentage of the group. Since almost all of these respondents indicated that they did masturbate, biological compensation was not the issue. On the other hand, 30.4% indicated frequent SRFOs "during periods of frequent waking orgasms or sexual arousal." Of course, some respondents selected BOTH of these conditions.

Survey Responses (n=200)
SFRO experiencers only
17f. During which of the following conditions have sleep-related orgasms been more frequent for you? Check all that apply.

  33% During the premenstrual stage of your monthly cycle
  16% During your menstrual flow
19.5% During the beginning of your monthly cycle, after your menstrual flow
   9% During pregnancy
 2.8% During nursing after giving birth
 8.6% During recovery from pregnancy
 8.6% During the beginning of menopausal Symptoms
   9% After menopause
14.3% At the beginning of new romantic relationship
 1.0% After death of spouse or sexual partner
30.4% During periods of frequent waking orgasms or sexual arousal
38.5% When between/ without, a sexual relationship
21.8% During periods of anxiety or worry

Other conditions mentioned by respondents:

 16% Can't tell/ haven't noticed
  2% During ovulation
  3% When meditating a lot/kundalini active
  3% When withdrawing from antidepressants or discontinuing birth control pills
  2% When flirting, feeling attractive/romantic
  2% Unwanted ending of a relationship
  1% During IVF treatments

Table 10 – Common Conditions Associated with SRFOs

Since some of the conditions listed on this table are age-dependent, it should be noted that many respondents age 40 or older mentioned menopause as a frequent condition associated with SRFOs. Pregnancy related conditions were frequently selected by those in the 20 thru 40s age ranges, but never even mentioned by those in the 50+ range. I included several items in this question related to the menstrual cycle because I had received so many anecdotal reports. This relationship has not been studied previously.

ACTIVE INCIDENCE THROUGHOUT THE LIFE SPAN

It is useful at this point to look at changes and peaks in SRFO responses throughout the lifespan. As indicated in Table Nine, 95% of my SRFOs experiencers had experienced SRFOs within the previous five years. Kinsey considered this to be the "active incidence" as opposed to the "accumulative incidence" or the total percentage of women who had ever experienced SRFOs. Kinsey, with his total sample of 7789 women regarding this topic, reported "only one instance of a female over seventy years of age who was having sex dreams to orgasm" (Kinsey et al. 1953, 200). My survey experiencers in the 70s-80s age range did not report an active incidence.

In Kinsey's data, the age decade with the peak active incidence was the age 40 to 50 range, with 22 to 38 percent of his sexual dreamers, depending on marital status, active in this period, and a declining rate in older age decades. Extrapolating, this would mean that 53 to 92 percent of his sleep orgasm experiencers were active in the decade from age 40 to 50. In my data, those in their 50s and 60s continued to be quite active. While this might be an effect of how I received survey responses (primarily internet), one would think that this effect would be the same for all age groups.

Survey Responses (n=174)
17a. Have you experienced a sleep-related orgasm during the past five years? (Yes responses by age):

Teens	100%
20-29	98%
30-39	100%
40-49	97%
50-59	91%
60-69	94%
70 & above	0%

Table 11 – Active Incidence of SRFOs by Age Decade

I asked my respondents to rate the age decades during which SRFOs were most common for them: first, second third.   While there was considerable individual variation, the overall pattern among my SRFO experiencers was to rate whatever age decade they were in as the most active. This was true for women in their 20s, 30s, 40s, 50s, and 60s, with slightly more variability for women in their 60s. In most cases, the overall pattern was for women to rate the preceding decade as the second most active period. So, of my experiencers, women in their 60s were somewhat split on whether SRFOs had been more common in their 50s or 60s.

Realistically, there were many *physiological* factors related to SRFOs that Kinsey's study did not address, especially the role of hormonal fluctuations. Nonetheless, he and his team provided far more information than had been previously available, and dispelled several myths. They also raised many questions. Since there were so many different factors contributing to this response, where should future researchers begin their investigation? And if biological compensation was not the cause, how should these occurrences be viewed morally? Both of these points have probably deterred many from pursuing further research.

> Something else that may be of interest to your study is that I have been struggling with vulvar vestibulitis and painful intercourse on and off for the past 3 years. At the onset of this condition is when I began to experience nocturnal orgasms. (age 22)

> I am abstinent and have not been sexually active in over two years. My SRFOs have been more frequent since becoming abstinent (7 in the last year). (age 24)

> They happen most often when I'm having lots of orgasms outside of dreaming, either through masturbation or sex. (age 30)

> They tend to occur either when I am having lots of sex and orgasms, or none at all. (age 30)

> When less sexually active. (age 32)

> But I have noticed nocturnal sleep orgasms occurring more frequently on the nights when I've had sex [always with no orgasm] before going to sleep. (age 33)

I noticed recently I have been having orgasms in my sleep but I wake up feeling good and happy. This has only been occurring in the last year more frequently. I'm not complaining :) but I'm just curious as to what makes it happen. I am 36 years old and have an active sex life with my boyfriend of 5 years. My boyfriend satisfies me all the time. (age 36)

Sex and intimacy with my spouse is very passionate and intense. We have been together for 11 years and I frequently have sexual dreams about my husband no matter what time of the month, and regardless of our level of activity and satisfaction. My orgasms are very intense from these erotic dreams and wake me up. There is no physical contact with my body during my dreams or orgasm from my dreams. (age 37)

When I've been around sexy men who are not my partner. (age 48)

I'm not completely comfortable telling you all of the following, but you are a clinical sexologist, so you might find it interesting. I am 40 years old. I have had sleep-related orgasms for as long as I can remember, so I assume that they started in puberty. I estimate that I have two of them a month, so I was a little surprised to read that "fewer than 10 percent of women...report having nocturnal orgasms more than five times a year." If my estimate of two per month is correct, and if I've been having them since I was, say, 12, I have had 672 of them. I wonder if this is a record number of orgasms for a virgin! I guess I'm lucky. I've been having more lately (five in March, three so far in April). Maybe they're increasing because of my age; you said that Kinsey found that they peaked in the forties and fifties. (age 40)

I have more SRFOs periodically, and then less for awhile; they are not really regular. (age 47)

I have recently entered into a long distance relationship with a man who regularly sends highly erotic emails to me. I have noticed that instead of occasional orgasms in my sleep I am having 1-2 a week. This has really surprised me as menopause has really decreased my level of overall sexual desire and I have had considerable trouble achieving orgasm through self masturbation (even when drawing on my partner's erotic prose). (age 49)

During a time when my waking sexual experiences have been less than satisfying, I find that I will have a sleep related orgasm. (age 54)

I am a 67 year old female. I live happily alone. I have not been in any kind of sexual relationship for over 20 years, but I occasionally have srfos. (age 67)

The System Check Theory

This has been the dominant theory since Kinsey's time, and while it has some merits, it really does not cover most of the realities. This theory implies that the body experiences these sleep-related orgasms "simply [as] a check to make sure a person's brain, nervous system, and genitals are healthy and in good working order." (Reinisch 1990, 89) This idea falls apart rather quickly when one considers that many women never experience these at all regardless of their circumstances. Overall, it implies a function and a regularity (or randomness) that simply is not supported by the available evidence.

NEWER UNDERSTANDINGS

As noted, Kinsey focused primarily on the psychological and behavioral causes of SRFOs. Since then, we have learned so much about possible physiological causes of SRFOs, especially the roles of hormones, the neurophysiology of the human sleep cycle, the stages of orgasm, effects of general physiological stimulation of the human nervous system, and the operation of the brain. Some women today think that sexologists have gone too far in "medicalizing" discussions of female sexuality, that science moves too quickly to classify situations as disorders or dysfunctions. Regardless of classifications, I think it is important to understand our basic physiology. I discussed some of the current ideas about the female nervous system as it relates to orgasm in Chapter Seven. I am going to begin this segment on *Newer Understandings* by discussing some of the other physiological influences on SRFOs. In Chapter Three, I mentioned that SRFOs are associated with the REM stage of sleep, so I'll start this part of the discussion by talking more about the human sleep cycle.

Brain Activity During Sleep

THE HUMAN SLEEP CYCLE

In recent years we have learned much more about how our brains function, including how they function during sleep. During sleep, brainwaves, recorded by electroencephalograms (EEG), tend to move through regular cycles lasting around 90 minutes each which repeat throughout the night. The REM (Rapid Eye Movement) stage is the last phase of this cycle, and grows longer towards morning. In the REM phase of sleep, our brains are actually 50 to 200 times more active than while we are awake or in deep sleep, even though our voluntary muscles are paralyzed (NIH). It is during this REM stage that both male and female genitals engorge, and during which SRFOs usually occur. The REM stage is also strongly associated with learning and dreaming, although some less vivid dreams do occur in stage two of NREM (Non-Rapid Eye Movement) sleep as well. Today some sleep researchers are viewing brain activity during REM as similar to the "scan and defrag" functions on our physical computers, with the resultant realignments of information leading to greater creativity and efficiency (Kluger 2012). Regardless of what is actually happening, we know that REM sleep is necessary for emotional health and well-being.

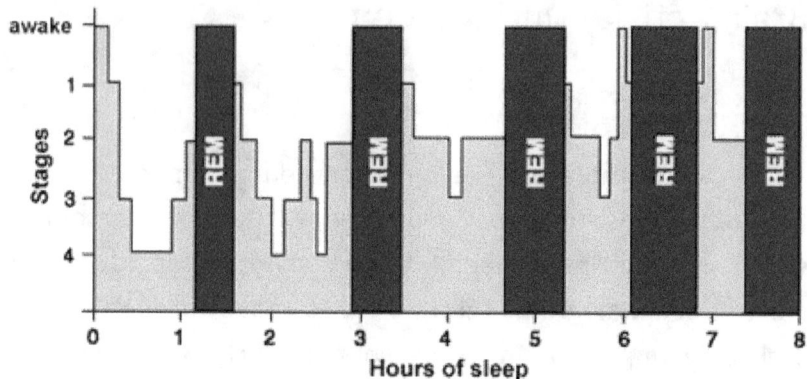

Fig. 2 – Stages of the Human Sleep Cycle (NIH-Adptd from Dement (1976)

The NREM phase consists of four stages, with very slow brain waves predominating in the beginning of the night. Overall, the NREM periods becomes shorter as the night progresses. It appears that physiological regeneration is an important function of the NREM phase.

Each stage of sleep is necessary for our survival and health. As adults, we spend about 20% of our sleep time in REM, or about 100-120 minutes each night. As young infants, we need about 16 hours of sleep each day, and spend about 50% of our sleep time in REM. Our overall need for sleep decreases gradually as we age, and the proportion of time spent in REM also changes. While the proportion of sleep which occurs in REM decreases until age 13 or so, it actually increases again in the 14-30 ages ranges, before starting to decrease again. See Figure 3.

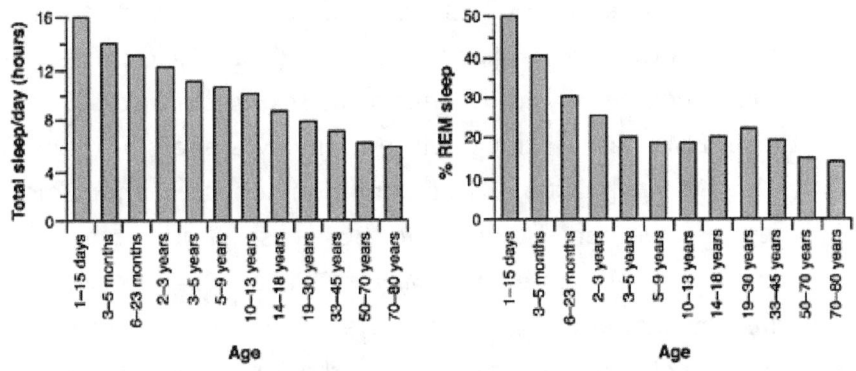

Data from Roffwarg, H.P., J.N. Muzio, and W.C. Dement. 1966. Ontogenetic development of the human sleep-dream cycle. *Science*, 152: 604–619.

Figure 3- Fluctuations in Duration of Sleep and REM periods by age

Typically, during the NREM phase, sleepers have no awareness at all and their voluntary muscles are NOT paralyzed. There are many differences between REM and NREM sleep, including differences in sexual responses. There are also specific sleep dysfunctions unique to the REM or NREM phases of sleep.

SLEEP DISORDERS RELATED TO SEX

1. Sexsomnia

Due to a dysfunction in the normal brain wave sequencing of the sleep cycle, some people experience sleep disorders (parasomnias) like "night terrors," sleep-walking, sleep-talking, sleep-eating, or even sleep-driving during NREM sleep. In these episodes, they move around and appear to be awake, and yet have no awareness of themselves or memory of what they do. It is very difficult to wake someone up during these incidents.

In the early 2000s, sleep researchers recognized a new sleep disorder now called "sleep sex" or "sexsomnia," in which people physically engage in *sexual behaviors* during the NREM phase of sleep, without any awareness or memory at all (Mangan 2005). This condition tends to affect more men than women. However, in these cases, both women and men are often more physically active and aggressive than when awake, and often vocalize extensively. For women, it usually includes very active masturbation, moaning, and/or initiating interaction with a bedmate (fondling, oral sex, intercourse). Sometimes sexsomnia includes a high incidence of paraphilic behaviors, which can lead to physical risk or even broken bones (Guilleminault et al. 2002). In extreme cases, it can include leaving the bedroom or home to seek a sexual partner, and might even include sexual assault. Sexsomnia has been successfully used as a legal defense. Again, it is very difficult to make someone wake-up when they are in this state.

In mild cases, with a willing partner, sexsomnia might not be a problem. Nevertheless, many of those who experience sexsomnia **do** suffer emotional problems as a result: feeling very frightened, confused, disbelieving, and ashamed when told about their behavior (Mangan 2004). Needless to say, sexsomnia can also lead to relationship problems.

Sexsomniacs usually have a history of other sleep disorders as well, especially sleep-walking. The prevalence of this disorder is really unknown; however, Mangan estimates that as much as 1% of the population might experience this. In one Canadian study of people with diagnosed sleep disorders, almost 7% had sexsomnia in addition to other sleep disorders.

Some researchers think that poor sleep habits, recreational drug use, and some of the pharmaceutical drugs used to induce sleep, might be contributing to its occurrence. It is best for people with this condition to consult a sleep therapist. In most cases, sexsomnia can be successfully treated with healthy sleep schedules, appropriate drugs, and/or CPAP machines to assist with nighttime breathing.

While sexsomniacs engage in sexual *behaviors*, orgasm is not a defining element. However, from several reports which I have received or read online, it appears that orgasms can occur during episodes of sexomnia...at least for men. One of my female correspondents has indicated that she thinks she experiences orgasm during sexsomnia based on reports from her husband. To date, I have not found any references to NREM orgasms for women happening while being monitored in a sleep lab. These orgasms are different than the REM-state SRFOs which are discussed throughout this book which typically do *not* include sexual *behaviors* due to muscle paralysis. It is also clear to me that some online writers are lumping REM-state orgasms into their discussions of sexsomnia.

2. Epilepsy

Another brain dysfunction which can generate orgasms during sleep is an epileptic seizure (Calleja, et al. 1988). Orgasms are sometimes generated by seizures in waking states also. Normally, women are aware when this happens during sleep. Orgasms during seizures are more common when the hypothalamus part of the brain is involved (Ruff 1980), and both waking and sleeping seizures can be controlled with anti-epileptic drugs.

3. Sleep Paralysis

There is another sleep disorder which can possibly impact the subjective interpretation of SRFOs, particularly in regard to "demons." Called "sleep paralysis" or SP, it is caused by a slight "glitch" or "hiccup" in the brain wave sequencing. This is an anomalous REM state condition which "consists of a period of inability to perform voluntary movements either at sleep onset (called hypnogogic or predormital form) or upon awakening (called hypnopompic or postdormital form)" (Dement 1999). If it happens at the beginning of sleep, the brain bypasses the NREM stages of the sleep cycle. As mentioned above, during REM sleep the brainstem turns off the sleeper's motor abilities and much sensory input. In sleep paralysis, this happens while the sleeper is still conscious or awake, and often able to open their eyes. If it happens upon awakening, awareness can return before the REM-state paralysis of the voluntary muscles has released.

There is some debate about whether SRFOs can actually occur during sleep paralysis due to its typically frightening nature. Female orgasms do not require motor abilities as shown by Holstege's PET scan research (2005), and as discussed in Chapter 6. Sleep orgasms usually occur *during* the REM stage as shown by Stephen LaBerge (1983), and other researchers when voluntary muscle paralysis is present. Several of my respondents mentioned that they sometimes experience sleep paralysis, but none indicated that they experience orgasms during those episodes.

Sleep paralysis usually only lasts a few seconds or minutes. Nonetheless, it can be quite disorienting, and often frightening, because the returning awareness often includes fragments of dream-state hallucinations mixed with elements of the physical surroundings. In addition, because voluntary muscle control is not active, it is not possible to intentionally move or take a deep breath. People often report the feeling of pressure on their chest, as if someone is sitting on them. No one is known to have ever died from SP; but the subjective experience might feel like impending death (Dement 1999). The perception of "pressure or pushing on the body may be so intense that the person feels as though s/he is being pushed or pulled into the bed" (Cheyne 2001, 146).

> In some cases, when the hypnogogic hallucinations are present, people feel that someone is in the room with them, some experience the feeling that someone or something is sitting on their chest and they feel impending death and suffocation. That has been called the "Hag Phenomena" and has been happening to people over the centuries. These things cause people much anxiety and terror, but there is no physical harm. (Dement 1999)

The hallucinations are not always terrifying. In some cases they are experienced as profoundly spiritual, and for some, they have constituted a spiritual awakening with life-changing insights. (Cheyne 2001).

Scientists are investigating many different ideas as to why sleep paralysis occurs, and the mechanisms by which the experience of a "sensed presence" is so consistent. Sleep Paralysis seems to be familial; however, it is not known whether it is a function of genetics or environmental factors. Michael Persinger of Laurentian University (1987) has demonstrated that the sensed presence phenomenon in waking states is associated with the impact of weak electromagnetic field patterns on neural synapses, especially around the temporal lobes of the brain. He contends that people are exposed to these daily in a variety of ways, including proximity to electrical power lines and geo-physical events like earthquakes.

In recent years, many researchers have attributed a variety of paranormal and spiritual experiences to the sensed presence phenomenon, usually as it occurs in sleep paralysis, since so many reports are associated with sleep or relaxation. Currently this is a significant component of the scientific explanations for experiences or perceptions of incubi/succubi contacts (Hufford 1982; Cheyne, 2001; Deane 2003; Conesa 2004; and others). Some people who experience SP frequently can train themselves to convert these experiences into lucid dreams or more pleasurable encounters (Conesa 2000).

Sometimes the sensed presence is attributed to something or someone other than a ghost or demon. For example:

> I used to think my step dad was touching me in my sleep ... but I can successfully rule that out now. (age 21)

Hormonal Fluctuations

The role of hormonal fluctuations is rarely addressed in regard to SRFOs. Nonetheless, many women notice this connection rather easily, and it is certainly one of the most dominant factors. Obviously, we know so much more about hormones today than Kinsey did sixty years ago.

When I asked survey participants about the conditions during which SRFOs were most common, they frequently identified periods of hormonal fluctuations. Puberty is obviously recognized as a period of hormonal change specifically related to sexual development. As noted in earlier chapters, many young women begin to experience SRFOs during this time. Likewise, various stages of the menstrual cycle, pregnancy, and menopause are frequently mentioned as periods of increased SRFO frequency. See Table 10.

PUBERTY

In the United States, girls are entering puberty at earlier ages than in the past. In 1999, the "normal" age range for breast development was lowered to age 8; however, cases of "precocious puberty," earlier than age 8, are still increasing. Researchers are very actively studying many different possible causes for this. There is a strong connection between obesity and early sexual development. "The single best predictor for the onset of menarche is weight, which is approximately 106 pounds when menarche begins" (Colburn, et al 1996, Moffitt et al. 1992).

Some researchers attribute the higher weights to lifestyle issues like fast food and less exercise. Others see both the weight gain and early sexual development as by-products of foods which have been contaminated with excessive hormones, i.e., dairy, beef, chicken, or consumption of too many soy products which contain natural estrogens. Others point to environmental chemicals like pesticides, or exposure to chemicals in common products like plastics. And still others point to the influence of cultural factors.

Whatever the cause, it is likely that earlier sexual development is also leading to the earlier onset of SRFOs, and the increased reports of "first orgasms" in this manner as described in Chapter Five.

There are so many different hormones that affect our lives and our sexuality. I am not an endocrinologist, so I am not going to attempt to discuss this in depth. However, I do want to point out a few connections that probably have a specific impact on incidence of sleep orgasms. Perhaps this will encourage others to investigate further.

During sleep, the brain produces, or signals the release of, a wide variety of neurotransmitters and hormones designed to regulate growth, health, and various bodily cycles, including the circadian rhythms of sleep itself.

> Sleep is one of the events that modify the timing of secretion for certain hormones. Many hormones are secreted into the blood during sleep. For example, scientists believe that the release of growth hormone is related in part to repair processes that occur during sleep. **Follicle stimulating hormone** and **luteinizing hormone**, which are involved in maturational and reproductive processes, are among the hormones released during sleep. In fact, the sleep-dependent release of luteinizing hormone is thought to be the event that initiates puberty. Other hormones, such as thyroid-stimulating hormone, are released prior to sleep. (NIH)

LUTEINIZING HORMONE

Luteinizing hormone (LH) is secreted from the anterior pituitary gland in varying quantities at different stages of the menstrual cycle. It is normally secreted during sleep in pulses, about once an hour. In addition to initiating puberty, a large "LH surge" each month signals ovulation to occur. During pregnancy, levels of hCG, a hormone very similar to LH, remain high. Levels of follicle stimulating hormone (FSH) and LH also increase significantly during menopause, and LH levels remain higher during the post-menopausal years. These are all times when SRFOs are frequently reported.

Luteinizing hormone (LH) undoubtedly plays a large role in the generation of SRFOs, because it plays a major role in the reproductive functions of both men and women in general. In men, LH signals the production of testosterone. In women, LH plays a more complex role. We know that it signals the release of an egg which leads to production of androstenedione, estrogen, and a low level of testosterone. It also signals the creation of a corpus leatum and consequently higher progesterone levels.

Unfortunately, I have not seen any research regarding the role of androgens, estrogens, or LH on female genital engorgement during sleep or sleep orgasms specifically. We know that male nocturnal erections depend on androgens (testosterone), but waking male erections depend more on dopamine (Montorsi and Oettel 2005). We know that when teen boys are given testosterone for therapeutic reasons, nocturnal emissions increase (Finkelstein et al. 1998).

Many years ago, renowned sex therapist Helen Singer Kaplan in her book *Disorders of Sexual Desire* (1979) noted that estrogen did not increase sexual desire in women, and testosterone was the hormone of "desire" for both men and women. Since then, testosterone has been used to treat women with low sexual desire, with very mixed results. Kaplan also hypothesized that LH itself might be a more effective treatment for low sexual desire for women. LH and testosterone both increase during waking female sexual arousal (Exton et al. 1999).

Some women report a reduction in sexual desire while taking birth control pills. Typically, birth control pills block the LH surge which signals ovulation to occur. Interestingly, some of my survey respondents report fewer SRFOs when they are taking birth control pills.

Recently, Swiss fertility researcher, Michel Jemec, has been studying the role of LH in sexual desire and applied for a U.S. patent on a new kind of synthetic LH drug (2009) to enhance sexual desire. He calls LH the "life hormone" and thinks it is responsible for overall levels of drive, motivation and energy (libido). According to him, LH levels are often higher in sportswomen and high achievers. Currently a synthetic version of LH (Luveris) is used in some fertility treatments including Invitro Fertilization (IVF) to induce ovulation. Jamec's research notes that it can cause spontaneous orgasms without touch (Talbot 2011). There are several internet message boards for women who are undergoing IVF and other fertility treatments to stimulate ovulation that contain numerous reports of SRFOs.

High LH levels are also associated with menopausal hot flashes, although a direct cause and effect relationship has not been established. This is a stage during which many women report an increase in SRFOs, despite the fact that the quality of both sleep and dreaming is often reduced.

Although other hormones and neurotransmitters are probably involved, I think LH merits much greater study in relationship to SRFOs

> I am currently breastfeeding and have not had any wet dreams since the birth of my daughter. Usually I have them pretty frequently. (age 21)

> I don't remember having them until after I had my daughter [...] Until recently I remember dreaming about having orgasms, but in the past few months I have been waking up in the middle and at the end of an orgasm. I had one last night and when I wake up after having them I immediately have the urge to go back to sleep...I have had these SRFO'S up to 5 times a night...I experience very long orgasms anyway so having up to 5 orgasms a night in my sleep, the length that I do have them, may start to cause some problems. I'm not too worried at this point, because i'm not going to say i don't enjoy them, but I would like to see some more research on them. (age 23)

> I have only had an orgasm during dreams [...] I may have had an orgasm or two during my last pregnancy and nursing period, though I am not positive. I am pregnant now, and the dreams are beginning again. I am afraid that I will never have an orgasm while awake, and that after my pregnancy and nursing period is over, I will not have the dreams either. (age 23)

> I think they are more frequent when I am off the pill. [I have had SRFOs] for the last 7 years

like clockwork on days 17-18 of my menstrual cycle...but have recently gone back on the pill and am not having them now. (age 31)

I experienced sleep orgasms mostly after IVF treatment. (age 34)

I think it's great that you asked at which point in the menstrual cycle do these orgasms tend to occur. I find that mine have tended to happen the week immediately prior to my period. (age 36)

It just happens all during the month at all times during my cycle. But I do feel aroused more when I'm on my period. (age 41)

More frequently for me during ovulation- increase in mucus and desire! (age 55)

I have had SRFOs for the last two nights in a row. I am going through Paxil withdrawal this week, the symptoms of which have been pretty uncomfortable, and which seem to be triggering my sexual response in the sense that I have not felt sexual or "horny" in a long time and this week I am feeling that way. I am attributing it to the withdrawal symptoms. (age 55)

Over this time period [when experiencing SRFOs] I was peri-menopausal. Once into and through menopause, intensity waned in all areas. I concluded that hormones act on women like mind-altering drugs. (age 63)

Why I looked it up this morning is because I had one last night. As far as I can remember I had no sexual stimulation during the day....I was scraping paint off an old door all day...no major interaction with anyone...didn't even watch TV, read my book, but nothing sexual (sound pretty boring, doesn't it?) As far as I know it came out of the blue. Before menopause I used to have a lot more. Unfortunately, they are pretty infrequent these days. (age 67)

OXYTOCIN

Oxytocin (OT) is another hormone and neurotransmitter which undoubtedly plays a major role in SRFOs. OT regulates numerous physiological aspects of sex, including the release of LH. Since the beginning of the 20th century, it has been recognized as the hormone which causes contractions during childbirth, the nursing/lactation reflex, and more recently, the contractions of orgasm.

In recent years, the strong *emotional* effects of OT have been more widely recognized. Because of this, several authors now use the phrase, "the Big O" to refer specifically to Oxytocin (Robinson 2009). Sometimes known as the "cuddling hormone," the "love hormone," or the "trust hormone," it acts to stimulate emotional bonding during pregnancy, childbirth, nursing, and partnered sex, and increases feelings of well-being after masturbation. It also increases romantic feelings and sense of security around a mate, reducing feelings of anxiety and fear.

The effects also extend to more ambiguous social situations, reducing social anxiety and increasing empathy and group bonding. "Administration of oxytocin (OT) can enhance trust, empathy and a host of other pro-social feelings" (McNamara 2011; MacDonald and MacDonald, 2010).

Produced in the hypothalamus and stored in the posterior pituitary gland, oxytocin can be administered therapeutically in several forms, most commonly as a nasal spray. It has been popular in Europe for treatment of various sexual dysfunctions and some psychological disorders. Since oxytocin levels tend to decrease with age, it is often used with older couples. Its use has not yet caught on as much in the United States as a treatment modality; however, OT has been receiving much more press.

Oxytocin also plays a significant role in regulating sleep, and perhaps even dream *content*. Patrick McNamara writes:

> Levels of oxytocin peak at around 5 hours after sleep onset when REM sleep predominates....
>
> Take the fascinating case of sex in dreams. Everyone has experienced dreams of sexual contact and even orgasm due to a dream of sexual contact with someone we love or desire. Now in normal waking life oxytocin is the hormone that mediates orgasm. It is very likely it does so in dreams as well. Then there is the fact that REM sleep is consistently associated with erections in males and clitoral engorgement in females. In waking life oxytocin is crucial for these physiologic responses. It seems likely that OT would

mediate such responses in dreams as well. (McNamara 2011)

Could it really be possible that hormones determine the *content* of our dreams? While this a rather controversial idea, current research is suggesting that brain chemicals might play a much larger role in the content of sleep cognitions that had previously been thought. We will look at dreams in more detail in the next chapter.

CORTISOL

Another hormone receiving much more research attention regarding its role in human sexual response is cortisol. Cortisol is produced by the adrenal glands. For many years it has been known as the "stress" hormone. In recent years it has gained a reputation as the "belly fat" hormone. The release of cortisol is signaled by the hypothalamus through the pituitary gland, and one of its main roles is to restore/maintain system homeostasis or balance. Cortisol levels have a huge effect on many parts of the body including metabolism, the immune system, bone development and health, skin health, kidney functions and other fluid excretions, blood pressure, and the reproductive system. Cortisol also effects memory and moods.

We know that cortisol levels rise in stressful or anxious situations, often as a result of attitudes and interpretations regarding the situation. Cortisol levels build more slowly and linger longer than those of its well-known companion, adrenaline. For women, testosterone is produced in both the ovaries and the adrenal glands. Persistently high OR low cortisol levels due to chronic stress reduce testosterone production (and consequently sex drive) for both men and women.

The effects of short-term fluctuations are less clear. Recent research has attempted to determine the effects of rising cortisol levels during female sexual *arousal*. So far the results have been somewhat mixed, so more research is needed to determine the specific factors that influence this response and what effect it might have (Hamilton et al. 2008, Goldey and van Anders 2011). In general, it appears that sexual intercourse and orgasm reduce cortisol levels.

Later in this chapter I will discuss the role of anxiety and pre-sleep sexual arousal as they relate to SRFOs; however, for now I will mention that cortisol may have a special relationship to SRFOs. Cortisol levels tend to fluctuate over a twenty-four hour period. In a healthy person, the lowest levels in the blood and urine occur around midnight, or an hour or two after falling asleep, when NREM is dominant. Cortisol levels increase significantly as morning approaches, when REM states predominate in the sleep cycle. There is an additional cortisol surge about a half hour after awakening. While there is some variation among individuals, most people have a fairly consistent personal cycle. Research regarding cortisol changes throughout the menstrual cycle has shown mixed results (Kudielka and Kirschbaum 2003; Nepomnaschy et al. 2011).

Some researchers, like cognitive neuroscientist Jessica Payne at Notre Dame University, have recently suggested that the higher cortisol levels during these close-to-morning REM stages of sleep might contribute greatly to the process of consolidating learnings, finding resolutions to problems, identifying creative solutions, and basically re-assembling or re-organizing the material that has been stirred up or "defragged" during the electrically active REM states (Kluger 2012). Sleep orgasms seem to have a role in restoring system homeostasis and, in this context, might represent a kind of creative solution or effective reorganization. It seems likely that early morning cortisol could facilitate that happening. On the other hand, it might simply be contributing to overall arousal levels.

DOPAMINE

Since I am discussing brain chemicals, I will include here a few words about dopamine, a neurotransmitter rather than a hormone, which strongly affects both waking and sleep-related orgasms. It is often mentioned in regard to waking sex because of its role in regulating pleasure-driven behavior and motivation. It makes us feel *happy*, euphoric, elated, and exhilarated. Dopamine is now recognized as the chemical responsible for feelings of "being in love" as well as sex and love addictions.   Rewards, whether physiological or psychological, increase the dopamine levels in our brains. It plays a major role in waking male erections, and female arousal as well. It is sometimes said that dopamine brings us together; but oxytocin keeps us together.

Dopamine is often implicated in addictive behaviors as people seek to maintain high levels in their systems. In addition, some addictive drugs, like cocaine, methamphetamine, and even nicotine, directly affect the dopamine centers in the brain.   Interestingly, recent anecdotal evidence suggests that one of the popular anti-smoking drugs, varenicline, which blocks the dopamine rewards of nicotine, also reduces the intense sexual arousal symptoms of Persistent Genital Arousal Disorder (PGAD) (Korda et al. 2009)

Dopamine also significantly impacts cognition or awareness. It *focuses our attention,* at times to the point of obsession. In recent years, it has been shown that the *experience* of dreaming, or *awareness* of dreaming, is totally dependent on the dopamine pathways and levels of dopamine in the brain, rather that the brainwave patterns of REM sleep, or neural connections to the brainstem pons. (Solms 1999). So, while OT might play a role in influencing the content of our dreams, dopamine allows us to be aware of them. We will explore dreaming further in the next chapter.

Although these chemicals affect our experiences, the connections between many chemical surges and our thoughts, desires, emotions, attitudes, and intentions are not well understood. Some of the discussion is similar to the question, "Which comes first, the chicken or the egg?" Do these chemicals of the brain cause us to think, feel, and behave in certain ways? Or do our thoughts, desires, fantasies, etc., cause the chemical changes in our brains? In the case of dopamine, oxytocin, cortisol, and even LH, there is definitely some interplay, and interactions can occur in both directions. In other words, we can influence the levels of these chemicals through our cognitive and behavioral choices.

Almost everyday, TV, magazine and internet articles offer tips on healthy ways to do this, including sunlight, exercise, and food choices. Simply pausing to think about, and make a quick list of, favorite pleasures or things for which we are grateful, increases dopamine levels. If some of our favorite pleasures or gratitudes include kind and loving relationships, we can increase our OT levels also. Just talking about sex increases LH levels in men which leads to

110

testosterone production (LaFerla et al. 1978). Thinking about a positive sexual experience (or writing a love letter) can increase testosterone levels in women (Goldey and van Anders 2011). And while we are all familiar with the rapid adrenaline rushes of the fight or flight response, the companion build up of cortisol is more sustained. These changes can all happen very quickly. This is probably why so many women are able to generate orgasms through fantasy alone.

Today, many scientists are studying the roles of hormones and neurotransmitters which impact sexual responses. This is one reason why it is often said that the brain is the greatest sex organ. This may be true, but increasingly we are learning that often the brain appears to be simply a transducer, responding to the elements of consciousness itself...our thoughts, attitudes, desires, imaginations, anticipations, fantasies, and memories...which operate this great sex organ.

Behavioral Factors

As noted previously, Kinsey found a slight positive correlation between sleep orgasms and masturbation, with or without accompanying fantasies. He also found that women who experienced frequent orgasms and multiple orgasms while awake, also experienced more sleep orgasms. He attributed this mostly to memory and imagination. Today, we recognize that for many women there is lingering physical arousal after sex, in addition to psychological arousal, whether or not orgasm has occurred (Sherfey 1972). Some writers recommend masturbation before sleep as a way to induce SRFOs. As mentioned above, masturbation to orgasm can increase both dopamine and OT levels.

111

For many women, masturbation and fantasy are important, if not essential, behaviors for learning about their bodies and sexual responsiveness. Therefore, I am going to discuss them in more depth in Chapter Eleven. Once learned, masturbation is often the most reliable opportunity for orgasm in a woman's life (Hite 1976).

Women's attitudes toward masturbation have changed significantly since Kinseys's time, although even then, 58% of his female survey respondents were able to masturbate to orgasm vs. 75% of my survey respondents. My figure today is very close to Shere Hite's findings in 1976.

Since the 1990s, it has been recognized that masturbation today is often viewed as simply one more expression of sexuality by those who are **already interested in sex and sexual experience,** rather than as a compensatory tool for low sexual outlet. Those with higher rates of other sexual activity, also have higher rates of masturbatory practice and more positive attitudes toward it. "It is an activity that stimulates and is stimulated by other sexual behaviors... the more sex you have of any kind, the more you may think about sex and the more you may masturbate" (Michael et al. 1994, 165).

Barbara Well's 1986 study of 245 undergraduate and graduate college women (average age 22.7 years) did not show masturbation to be a predictor or correlate of SRFOs. Her in-depth statistical analysis showed that SRFOs were correlated with numerous cultural factors, but few of the behavioral factors investigated by Kinsey. Her study tested nine hypotheses and fifty-eight predictor variables. In contrast to Kinsey's research, some of the investigated factors which were shown NOT to be predictive of SRFOs included: sexual experiences, variety of sexual experiences, frequency of participation in 17 different sexual activities, age, marital status, religiosity, and frequency of sexual dreams. Apparently, there is some other condition at work here beyond the sexual behaviors themselves.

Cultural Factors

While the Wells study (1986) showed correlations between SRFOs and several cultural factors, it definitely raised the "chicken or the egg" question. While 37% of her group had experienced SRFOs, 35% had never even heard of them. Factors which WERE correlated with SRFOs included:

1. satisfaction with one's sex life
2. high levels of erotic responsiveness (arousal)
3. anxiety
4. *sexual liberalism*
5. *waking sexually excited from sleep*
6. *being familiar with the phenomenon of nocturnal orgasm*
7. *having a positive attitude toward nocturnal orgasms.*

According to Wells, the italicized items had the strongest predictive value. My current survey suggests that the four italicized items are probably correlated due to "after the fact" conditions rather than predictive possibilities. As shown in my current survey, 93% of experiencers of all ages FIRST learned about SRFOs by experiencing them, and 77% enjoy them (Chapter 2). This enjoyment suggests a "positive attitude" toward them, but occurs after experiencing them. Realistically, to date, most women who do not experience them, do not even know about them, and are therefore unlikely to have any attitude.

113

Regarding item #5, fully 94.5% of my survey respondents reported awakening from sleep "feeling sexually aroused," and 87% reported experiencing SRFOs. In my survey, of the 5.5% who reported that they never awaken from sleep "feeling sexually aroused," 64% reported experiencing SRFOs. Given the prevalence of this factor, it is probably not predictive, although it is obviously correlated.

Survey Responses (n=200)
8. Have you ever awakened from sleep feeling sexually aroused?
Yes   94.5%   No   5.5%
If yes, how often?
18%   Less than 10 times in life
46%   Several times each year
24%   Several times each month
6.5% At least once each week

Table 12 - Awakening from Sleep Sexually Aroused

Regarding item #4, 31.5% of my survey respondents described their attitudes toward sex as "very liberal;" 33.5% as "somewhat liberal;" and 22.5% as "moderate." Of the 12% who described their attitudes as "somewhat conservative" or "very conservative," 83% experienced SRFOs, and half of them reported enjoying them! There was a slightly higher percentage of this group, than the overall SRFO group, that reported feeling "worried" or "embarrassed" by SRFOs, but most simply indicated that they were "curious" as to why they happened. So, it appears that "sexual liberalism" was not a predictive factor for SRFOs among my respondents, although it might predict their reactions to these orgasms after the fact.

Survey Responses (n=200)

5. How would you rate your attitudes about sex?   Please check
      2.5% Very conservative
      9.5% Somewhat conservative
     22.5% Moderate
     33.5% Somewhat liberal
     31.5% Very liberal

Table 13 – Attitudes about Sex

Psychological Factors

ANXIETY AND AROUSAL

I am addressing these two factors together because they share many similarities from the perspective of the brain during sleep.

The main factor that the Kinsey and Wells studies agreed upon as predictive of SRFOs was "high levels of erotic responsiveness (arousal)." "Anxiety" was correlated with SRFOs in the 1976 Henton study of 774 college undergraduates, and in two earlier studies (Tapia, Werboff and Winokur 1958; Winokur, Guze, and Pfeiffer 1959) of 59 and 100 women diagnosed with mental illness (as reported in Wells 1986, 425). These last two studies used groups of patient populations. Given the lack of distinct categories of mental illness, and the fact that at that time SRFOs were still viewed by many as indicators of pathology, it is difficult to assess these results.

In my study, SRFO experiencers rated *both* anxiety and arousal as frequent conditions associated with SRFOs (See Table Ten). I did not, however, ask any questions which would allow me to compare anxiety or arousal levels between experiencers and non-experiencers.

In general, anxiety is a feeling of worry or fear, usually about a possible situation in the future. It has both psychological and physiological components, including somatic, emotional, cognitive and behavioral responses. It is considered to be a normal response to stressors, so sometimes people simply call it "stress." When it is excessive, it can become an *anxiety disorder*. Today, many people talk about sex as a way to relieve stress.

Sexual arousal, or excitement, also has psychological and physiological components, which include somatic, emotional, cognitive and behavioral responses. Physiologically, the responses in the autonomic nervous system are very similar between sexual arousal and anxiety. However, the cognitive interpretations are quite different.

Physiological Stimulation and Excitation Transfer

Throughout recent years, sexologists have debated the relationship between anxiety and sexual arousal. There are many situations in which anxiety interferes with sexual arousal and orgasm in waking states. But recently, researchers have more widely recognized that anxiety can also have a facilitative effect on sexual arousal. Many sexual fantasies, for example, include situations that might be considered anxiety-provoking. The difference lies in the cognitive interpretation and context.

Kinsey (1953) very astutely noted the physiological similarities between a variety of emotional states and sexual arousal [...] He also noted that of twenty-four sympathetic and parasympathetic elements of physiological sexual response, most can also appear during states of anger, fear, or epilepsy. Male ejaculation was included in this list; however, female orgasm was not (Kinsey et al. 1953, 704). Nonetheless, other researchers have recognized "anger orgasms" and "stress orgasms" in women (Heiman, 1976). According to Kinsey, "one might hypothesize that if certain of the physiologic elements were prevented from developing in a sexual response, or taken away from a sexual response, the individual might be left in a state of anger or fear...The fact that frustrated sexual responses so readily turn into anger and rage might thus be explained" (Kinsey et al. 1953, 704). He also noted that occasionally anger or fear develop into a true sexual response (King 2006, 134).

Because anxiety is often viewed as a barrier to sexual arousal and orgasm, Masters and Johnson (1970) emphasized sensate focus (touching) exercises and other anxiety reducing techniques. Most clinicians can easily point to cases where anxiety has played an inhibitory role in the sexual response cycle, especially waking female orgasm.

Nonetheless, the overall effect of anxiety is somewhat paradoxical on both the emotional and physiological levels. As described by Jack Morin, author of *The Erotic Mind*, it can actually act as an aphrodisiac: "Attraction + Obstacles = Excitement" (Morin 1995, 48-71).

> The relationship between anxiety and eroticism is intricate and paradoxical. If you are highly anxious in a sexual situation, your physical capacities for arousal or orgasm or both will

usually be short-circuited . . . However, to view anxiety solely as antithetical to arousal is to blind ourselves to a richer and more challenging reality: just as surely as anxiety can disrupt arousal, it can also create, focus, and intensify it. Depending on the situation and the individuals involved, anxiety is either an antiaphrodisiac or an aphrodisiac – occasionally both.

Anxiety intensifies arousal by contributing to a generalized state of physical excitation. All forms of excitement, sexual and nonsexual alike, increase muscular tension, blood flow, and heart and breathing rates. Consequently, your body responds similarly to anxiety-provoking and sexually arousing situations. For instance, some men and women spontaneously experience sexual arousal in a wide range of frightening situations, including everything from fights to roller-coaster rides to sexual assaults. (Morin 1995, 117-8)

In addition, many of the physical sensations associated with *limerence,* or falling in love, as identified by Dorothy Tennov (1979), are virtually identical to those associated with anxiety. Many of the thoughts and feelings are as well.

Since sexual arousal and anxiety are so closely related to each other physiologically, both showing physiological excitation, it is not at all surprising that both are high predictors of SFROs, regardless of our subjective interpretations.

One interesting theory that has gained more attention and research in recent years is called *excitation transfer.*

Excitation transfer theory, as first described by Zillman (1971), posits residual excitement from a previous arousing stimulus or situation may serve to intensify a later emotional state [...] Sympathetic nervous system arousal does not terminate abruptly with the cessation of the eliciting conditions, but . . . declines slowly . . . It is during this period of residual excitement that an individual who is exposed to a subsequent emotion-provoking situation may misattribute the residual excitement to their current situation. By doing so, their experience of the subsequent emotional state may be intensified. (Meston and Frohlich 2003, 537)

One of the leading researchers studying female sexual arousal today is Cindy Meston at the University of Texas at Austin. She has conducted many fascinating studies demonstrating variations of excitation transfer. In one study she showed that the physical excitation of exercise (bicycle riding) enhanced sexual arousal. In another, the excitement of riding a roller coaster enhanced the sexual attractiveness of potential partners (2003). This same effect has been observed by other researchers after thrill-seeking behaviors like bungee jumping, which also elevate dopamine levels.

Meston has also conducted interesting research regarding the ways in which women tend to assess sexual arousal subjectively, with or without corresponding physiological cues. Throughout the history of sexological research, women have not been very good at judging when their bodies are sexually aroused, and often physiological arousal does **not** seem to correlate with the subjective experience or interpretation of sexual arousal. Some researchers are investigating the possibility of training women to consciously recognize sexual arousal through techniques such as biofeedback.

So much of our experience of sexual arousal and eroticism is really subjective interpretation, despite what the chemicals and organs of our bodies are doing. As David Schulz, in his 1984 book *Human Sexuality*, points out "human sexuality is to an unknown extent a creation of the human mind..." (Schulz 1984, 215). This tendency to form our own interpretations complicates the distinctions between anxiety and arousal. For example, there is some evidence that highly educated career women experience greater anxiety, yet tend to interpret it as sexual arousal. In some cases they have developed "conditioned cognitive expectancy for sexual arousal" (Palace and Godzilla 1990) and may choose to use orgasm as an anxiety management tool consciously through masturbation and unconsciously through SRFOs. Conversely, given the difficulty that most women demonstrate in subjectively recognizing sexual arousal as such, it is possible that in some cases women interpret sexual arousal as anxiety, especially during the monthly premenstrual phase.

Healthy Homeostasis or Excitation Integration

Some sex researchers have noted that our bodies are likely to resolve excessive sexual arousal or tension through orgasms in sleep. It is thought that since the hypothalamus directs the activity of the autonomic nervous system, which includes the sympathetic and parasympathetic arousal responses, and is also responsible for regulating system homoeostasis, it would be natural to assume that the inhibition provided by sleep would facilitate resolution of this sympathetic nervous system arousal through orgasm. Masters, Johnson, and Kolodny suggest that this is true for both men and women regarding sexual arousal, though no specific mechanism is hypothesized:

> If there has been considerable excitement but orgasm has not occurred . . . there is sometimes a lingering sensation of pelvic heaviness or aching that is due to continued vasocongestion. This may create a condition of some discomfort, particularly if high levels of arousal were prolonged. Testicular aching ("blue balls") in men and pelvic congestion in women may be relieved by orgasms that occur during sleep. (Masters, Johnson, and Kolodny 1982, 76)

The next question which arises through this discussion is the extent to which *excitation transfer of anxious arousal,* or other psychological or physiological arousal (i.e., hormonal) contributes to sexual dream content and SRFOs. The possibility of this interpretive, psychological transfer, combined with the activation of the hypothalamus during physiological arousal, suggests that SRFOs may indeed play an important role in regulating system homeostasis in a very broad way, beyond the orgasmic discharge of *sexual energy* per se, as hypothesized in several earlier theories.

I call this the "Healthy Homeostasis Theory of SRFOs." It acknowledges an energy-balancing role, though not limited to the idea of sexual energy or sexual arousal. Simply put, this suggests that the nervous system, an electro-chemical communication system, will use orgasms as a method to discharge excessive excitation regardless of the source of the excitation. This then releases soothing chemical responses like OT, and also prolactin which will induce sleep. The idea

121

of biological homeostasis; i.e., the body's maintenance of consistent temperatures, has been recognized since the early twentieth century. In the 1970s, the idea of psychological homeostasis, with endocrine system responses, became popular. Since the hypothalamus regulates the homeostasis of other biological conditions, like temperature, and plays a major role in releasing orgasmic hormones (oxytocin), it seems reasonable to assume that system homeostasis is one way to view the function of orgasms in general and SRFOs specifically.

Another possible variation of this idea would be what I call the "Excitation Integration Theory of SRFOs." This theory allows the possibility that SRFOs are not just releasing excitation and returning one to the previous state of balance, but rather allowing incorporation and assimilation of more excitation and energy movement, resulting in a slightly expanded pattern of integration and balance. Multiple orgasms in a waking state often have this feel, like a wave pattern of going higher and higher into greater expansion and wholeness. In both cases, the outcome is physiological balance.

From survey respondents:

I once had a dream orgasm after sex, but it wasn't about my partner and it wasn't sexually arousing. I'm assuming it was just due to postsexual tension. Or something. (age 15)

I had my 3rd "wet dream". I remember the dream vividly. I won't go into detail, but it involved me having sex with a major love-interest in my life at the time. I was also really stressed out at the time because I had also recently began my menstrual cycle. The most recent one happened about a week ago. I had dozed off on the sofa and had a very detailed lucid dream about the man I'm currently sexually involved with. I woke up to find myself having an orgasm. I'm also under a bit of stress with college and life at home. (age 20)

All four times I had not been touching myself. And all four times, I guess you could say I was mildly stressed out. (age 20)

Lately, I've had a cluster of several in just a few days after a long period of not having any. I remember the first one this week occurring during a not particularly sexy dream. Lately, life is stressful with my husband searching for a new job so I haven't been sleeping well which I am guessing is why I have had more lucid dreams. They are powerful and afterwards, it is hard to fall asleep so I may prefer to be without them for awhile. (age 35)

This week has been quite stressful and the past couple months have been quite sex-less. I've had three lucid dreaming orgasms in the past four days. (age 35)

I'm very interested in reading about the link to anger and anxiety. It is counterintuitive to me that those emotions would be linked to an increase in SRFOs, but I have felt a lot of anxiety lately and have been having a lot of them. (age 40)

After experiencing several SRFOs, [my husband] sent me off to see a psychologist, who told me it was normal, and probably a response to stress more than anything else. (age 42)

I have only had a few SRFOs, but the most dramatic was shortly after I was diagnosed with breast cancer at age 43. I had not yet decided on my course of action and was weighing all of my options ranging from mastectomy to lumpectomy. During this period I had a really powerful dream. It was centered around female breasts: I was at a musical concert of some sort and began having sex with the lead singer who had beautiful breasts. All of the sex was centered on breasts and I awoke in the midst of the most powerful orgasm I have ever experienced. Even the sex in the dream was amazing, although I am not a lesbian and it was all with a woman. (age 46)

I have only recently confided in my therapist... after a personal illness, death of a love, loss of job. I have not been "bothered" by sleep-related orgasms for 5 years. All of a sudden- Wham! They are back with a vengeance. (age 51)

The inclination toward SRFOs are interesting as it relates to energy, energy build up, and the body's sensibilities to do something about these. I am glad the body knows, and has an innate wisdom concerning all things life. (age 54)

SPIRITUAL INTERESTS AND PRACTICES

My survey included questions about spiritual practices because of observations I have made over the years in my own life experience. Aside from being a psychotherapist, I am an ordained minister, and have also taught various meditation and consciousness expansion techniques for over thirty years.

Interestingly, I once read results of a small unpublished study in which LH levels increased significantly, within minutes, after women began a kundalini meditation exercise (Khalsa and Khalsa 1976). In the Eastern tradition, kundalini is the name given to the basic, universal, lifeforce energy which flows through the body and consciousness. It lies coiled at the base of the spine in the first "chakra," or energy center, until it is awakened and begins to flow through the spinal column to the head, resulting in greatly expanded awareness or consciousness. There are many other results and symptoms of kundalini awakening including sexual arousal at times. Western philosophies really do not have a synonym for this idea, although the term "kundalini" is being used more often in the West, and many attest to experiencing it.

Other studies have shown no change in LH levels with Transcendental Meditation (Stein and Oz 2004). I would love to see more research on the impact of various spiritual practices on hormone production.

I think this topic is interesting because I have noticed that the timing of women's menstrual cycles often change rather quickly with initial exposure to meditation. Numerous anecdotal reports mention an increase in sexual desire and responsiveness due to these practices. Some women, including some survey respondents, also reported an increase in SRFO activity after experiencing meditative states, yoga, shamanic journeys, energy-based martial arts, or religious conversion experiences. Of course, these are also "altered states of consciousness" as are orgasm, sleep, and dreams.

Many of the writers in the Tantric/Sacred Sex field address this topic. Kenneth Ray Stubbs describes many kinds of orgasmic experiences in meditation and shamanic journeying (Stubbs 2000). Genia Pauli Haddon, in *Uniting Sex Self & Spirit,* makes a connection between LH, menopausal hot flashes, meditation, awakening kundalini, altered consciousness, and body voltage polarity shifts (Haddon 1993, 142-147). In the internet version of her book, *The Biology of Kundalini* (2008), Jana Dixon mentions that "this 'LH surge' could be why kundalini increases at this time [during ovulation] in women."

Although spiritual practices can lead to increases in sexual arousal, the opposite of this situation is also true. Jenny Wade, author of *Transcendent Sex* (2004), provides survey research showing that sex can lead to transcendent experiences and spiritual awareness. Gina Ogden, author of *The Heart and Soul of Sex: Making the ISIS connection* (2006), presents survey research highlighting how desire for a spiritual connection often motivates women toward sexual behavior. Some authors attribute this feeling to the bonding hormone, oxytocin, This is important research, but not exactly new. Many pre-Christian practices in Western civilization emphasized this relationship, in addition to the varied practices of the East. For many in these disciplines and philosophies, sexuality and spirituality are one.

From survey respondents:

When I was younger, growing up in quite a religious household, I struggled with masturbation and there was often a lot of guilt that accompanied it. Instead of guilt or tension accompanying the [sleep] orgasm, it felt more akin to a spiritual experience. I always look back on those moments with a sense of awe and hope I will be able to experience something similar again. I have no idea what any contributing factors could have been, but am very curious. (age 20)

My experience occurred recently over two consecutive nights. I have been feeling a little anxiety and anger lately, so have been actively working on my inner self through spiritual meditation classes and Chinese natural medicine, i.e. acupuncture. I never thought it [SRFO] possible, therefore am a little stunned...so if you have any other information on the subject I would greatly appreciate guidance! (age 27)

I would say that my base chakra and chi has been stimulated – the Kundalini energy is flowing – and it's as though the dreaming orgasms have been unblocking energy so the chi can flow as it is being stimulated by the martial arts and dance classes. (age 44)

[More SRFOs] during periods of meditation practice where it seems to also result in making it easier to be aware while dreaming, and that fuzzy state between awake and just before full sleep becomes very extended. (age 48)

I have noticed [...] when [in meditations] that I am sometimes very intensely aroused. Not all the time, but at least 10-20% of the time, I will have that reaction. It is not connected to any images or visualizations, but is jus a very erotic, sensual, horny feeling. It feels wonderful to relax into it. (age 53)

All of this [SRFOs] started when I went through a very powerful and emotional conversion experience. (If you're an atheist or otherwise skeptical, that's ok; just call it a powerful and emotional love experience with an imaginary Friend...) In any case, I was receiving spiritual direction at the time and shared all this with my spiritual director. His response was that it's not uncommon for men or women to experience arousal during an experience of the love of God, that our whole bodies sometimes respond to it. The thing was, though, that once it started, it didn't stop. I was in a state of very localized genital arousal 24 hours a day, 7 days a week. (age 56)

EDUCATION AND INTELLIGENCE

Regarding my survey respondents, it is difficult to draw too many conclusions based on education because they are not a representative sample of women at large. Obviously, they were a curious group, motivated and intelligent enough to find my web page and complete the survey. Because of the age spread, 15 to 85, the level of education varied from high school diplomas or less (11.5%) to doctoral degrees (5.5%), with 52% having a bachelor degree or higher. Many respondents were students, regardless of their ages or other circumstances. Overall, the level of education continued to increase throughout the age span resulting in 35% of respondents in the 60-79 age range holding doctoral degrees. All but two respondents in this age group had experienced SRFOs within the previous five years.

Now, having said that I do not want to draw too many conclusions, I found it interesting that 100% of respondents with doctoral degrees had experienced SRFOs at some point during their lives, and 91% of those with masters degrees had experienced SRFOs at some time in their lives. Remember, these percentages cannot be generalized to the population at large.

Kinsey noted, with some surprise, that sex dreams and nocturnal emissions were more common among educated men. "The males who go furthest in their educational career appear to have better developed imaginative capacities, and this seem to have an effect upon the development of their psychosexual responses" (Kinsey et al. 1953 201-2). He denied this connection in his narrative about women; however, his data clearly showed a connection for the most highly educated women.

From large sexological surveys over the past thirty years or so, we have learned that formal education has a tremendous impact on women's sexuality. Since so many survey respondents indicated an interest in this relationship, I am going to excerpt a segment from my first book which addresses education and related personality factors:

While the impact of education on the incidence or frequency of SRFOs has not been adequately studied, it would seem that there is a logical connection. Education provides exposure to many diverse ideas, as well as stimulation and development of the creative and discriminative mental faculties. The milieu of campus life during an important psychosexual developmental stage provides abundant opportunity for experimentation and exploration. Educational differences show up in sexual behavior throughout the lifespan, with more highly educated women continuing sexual activity into an older age (Janus and Janus 1993, 321). Kinsey's data showed this to be true of SRFOs also with the highly educated ("17+" years) group being the only single women educational level category to continue SRFOs past age forty (Kinsey et al. 1953, 218), and SRFOs representing a higher percentage of sexual outlet for highly educated women at all age levels, especially above age 35 (Kinsey et al. 1953, 563). "Those with more education – most dramatically, the women in the postgraduate group – showed a greater ability to make choices and to enjoy a more varied diet of sexual experience . . . they report much greater gratification in their sexuality" (Janus and Janus 1993, 321).

Higher education has a life-long impact on sexual attitudes, behavior, waking experience, imagination, motivation, and arousal. This might be sufficient to trigger SRFOs at a rate in excess of that experienced by less educated women. This is an untested hypothesis. The specific nature of the connection is unclear. Do well-educated women think about sex more than the less educated? If one is thinking about sex when awake, it is likely that sex will also appear in sleep-time mentations and images according to empirical research about dreaming. Are well-educated women more sexually aroused? Or does higher education have its impact by removing cultural myths and fears about experiencing sexuality?

Personality Factors

Underlying this behavioral data is the more basic issue of personality. Who are the women attracted to higher education to begin with? What qualities do they bring to the educational experience? What qualities to they seek to develop further? While the experience of formal education might contribute to SRFOs, it is also possible that the true predictors are personality characteristics that have not yet been studied at all in relationship to SRFOs. Chief among these would be self-confidence, competence, self-reliance, self-expression, creativity, assertiveness, adventurousness, and general tendencies toward self-actualizing, inner-directed motivation and generally good mental health.

Numerous studies since the 1930s have shown that women who rate highly on these personality factors are more orgasmic. Seymour Fisher, in his book Sexual Images of the Self (1989, 49-50) presents a good summary of these studies, and concludes by declaring "that active women are more effective in reaching orgasm than are passive women" (Fisher 1989, 50). Abraham Maslow, a humanistic personality theorist who studied happy, healthy, "self-actualizing" women in the 1930s-40s, was of the opinion that orgasmic sexual dreams are "characteristic of women who are self-assured, poised, independent and generally capable. Women with low self-esteem (who are more inhibited) usually have romantic, symbolic, anxious, or distorted sexual dreams, he found, compared to open dreams of the sexual act by women

131

with high self-esteem" (Maslow 1942, summarized in Garfield 1979, 126).

Given that incidence of SRFOs continues to increase with age, it is also possible that these experiences are products of a psychological maturation process which might lead to eventual development of the personality factors mentioned above, with or without formal education.

It also seems possible that SRFOs might be a basic indicator of intelligence. This notion comes from the fact that in Kinsey's sample, the women who eventually sought graduate school education often reported experiencing SRFOs at younger ages than less educated groups (Kinsey et al. 1953, 218). Higher education would not yet have taken place, and consequently the effects thereof would not yet have had an impact. Likewise, higher intelligence is often associated with the personality factors mentioned above. Fisher's discussion actually begins with mention of the famous Terman longitudinal study of 1300 high IQ children, which concluded that high IQ test scores were correlated with greater physical and mental health (Terman and Oden 1959). This is an interesting and totally untested hypothesis. (King 2006, 114-121)

A quick analysis of my current survey data does not show a specific correlation between advanced educational degrees and early onset of SRFOs. But as noted in Chapter Five, early onset was more common among my *entire* group of respondents than in Kinsey's group.

Chapter 10

What Do Dreams Have To Do with SRFOs?

Dreams have a lot to do with SRFOs, although the specific mechanisms by which they are related might vary more significantly than earlier hypothesized. Kinsey believed that "the dreams are not only necessary factors in the great majority of cases, but the prime precipitating factors of most nocturnal orgasms," although he did recognize that physiological factors could be influencing these as well (Kinsey et al. 1953 194). Data from my survey clearly suggests that dreams are not necessary, and actually, may NOT be the "prime precipitating factors." With the possible exception of lucid dreams, both the dreams and the SRFOs might be triggered by something else: the normal REM state functions, the pre-sleep state of physiological or psychological arousal (including anxiety), dopamine levels, LH pulses, or other hormonal fluctuations.

SEX DREAMS - FREQUENCY

Kinsey was very interested in "sex dreams" in general, and his body of research on this topic is still considered to be the most definitive. There simply has not been much research on sex dreams since then. It seems possible to me, however, that some of his interest in dreams might have skewed his thinking regarding SRFOs. In referring so consistently to "dreams with orgasm," his results might have left out too many reports of sleep-related orgasms without dreams! He reported only one percent of such orgasms without memory of dreams. By contrast, of my SRFO experiencers, 50% reported sleep orgasms without awareness of a preceding dream. Of course, 90% of experiencers reported times when SRFOs *were* preceded by an erotic dream; but 36% also reported times when the preceding dream was not erotic, sexy, or sensual. (See Chapter Five)

Kinsey estimated that 70% of women would experience a sexual dream during their lifetime; while almost 100% of men would. Beginning in the late 1970s to mid 80s, dream researchers began to notice that women were reporting sex dreams at almost the same rate as men, probably due to cultural factors: the sexual revolution, etc. (Kremsdorf et al. 1978; Robbins et al. 1985). In my current survey, 96.5% of women reported having an overtly sexual or erotic dream, and of the 3.5% who did not, most experienced SRFOs.

Survey Responses (n=200)

6. Have you ever had a dream that you would consider to be overtly sexual or erotic?

      Yes: 96.5%   No 3.5%

7. Have you ever had a dream in which you were having sex with someone else?

      Yes: 91.5%   No: 8.5%

If yes, how often:

      23.0% Less than 10 times in life
      47.0% Several times each year
      14.5% Several times each month
      6.5% At least once each week
      1.5% No estimate

Table 14 – Incidence of Erotic Dreams including Sex with Another

Survey Responses (n=200)
8. Have you ever had a sex dream in which you witnessed others having sex?
Yes: 46%   No: 54%
If yes, how often:
31.5% Less than 10 times in life
10.5% Several times each year
2.0% Several times each month
.5% At least once a week
1% No estimate

Table 15 – Incidence of Erotic Dreams Observing Others

As I said, there has been very little contemporary research about sexuality in dreams despite the genital arousal that occurs naturally during REM. For those who are interested, my first book includes a lengthy chapter which reviews then existing research. This book will simply highlight a few ideas, then focus on newer understandings from my survey and very recent research. For an in-depth look at the history of dreaming and dream research, I recommend *Our Dreaming Mind* (1994) by Robert Van de Castle, former director of the sleep lab at the University of Virginia, and still an international leader in the study of dreams.

THEORIES OF DREAMING

By way of background, it is probably useful to know that one of the big questions in dream research over the past hundred-plus years has been whether dream content is compensatory or continuous. This is the same question which had been raised regarding SRFOs.

1. Dreaming as a Psychological Process

The compensatory theory was popularized by Sigmund Freud in his classic, *The Interpretation of Dreams* (1900). Greatly simplified, Freud felt that in essence, all dreams were neurotic attempts at wish fulfillment driven primarily by sexual urges. The dreams were attempts to satisfy needs and wishes that were not being met in waking life. This idea that all dreams were essentially sexual and pathological probably stopped many from discussing their dreams at all. Of course, Freud felt that much of the imagery was symbolic; therefore, people required a trained psychoanalyst to help them understand the dream content.

Realistically, Freud's view was a big step forward from the previous opinion that the dreams of ordinary people were the evil work of the devil (See Chapter Nine). He brought dreams into public awareness. He also opened the door to the investigation of dream content and symbology. While many therapists, including Carl Jung, held on to the idea that dreams were compensatory; many rejected, modified, and/or expanded upon Freud's opinions.

2. The Empirical Dream Researchers

The empirical school of dream research emerged in 1953 when scientists, using EEG machines, first associated dreaming with the Rapid Eye Movement (REM) period of the normal ninety-minute sleep cycle (Aserinsky and Kleitman 1953). Armed with new technology, dedicated researchers observed, measured, recorded, and analyzed correspondences between physiology and dream reports. Many of these early empirical sleep and dream researchers were drawn into this field by their interest in Freudian concepts. Consequently, early researchers in this group also studied issues like genital engorgement or arousal during REM sleep.

Gradually, through the 1950s-80s, findings by the empirical researchers began to contradict many of Freud's theories. As the empiricists continued to gather data about dream content, it became clear that most dream content was rather mundane, directly related to experiences and images in current daily life. Consequently, opinion shifted to the idea that dream content is *continuous*; that it is basically a continuation of whatever is happening in daily life.

In addition, In 1962, research by Foulkes revealed that some kind of mental activity is always occurring through the night. The NREM mentations tend to be more like waking thinking, often with endless loops of repetitive thought. While NREM ideas *can* be very creative, the REM period experiences are more vivid, distorted, visual, detailed, multi-sensory, or hallucinatory, like a different reality. Nevertheless, since then, there has been a gradual breakdown in the close association between REM states and dreaming. Due to these NREM mentations, some dream and consciousness researchers (Flanagan 2000) now hold the opinion that dreams occur throughout the night, especially in stage 2 NREM. This is one of the current controversies in sleep and dream research (Dement 1992; Domoff 2001).

Comments by G. William Domhoff, a current dream content researcher at the University of California, provide a useful summary of the empirical school perspective.

> In short, a very large body of literature contradicts the claim that dreams are difficult to decipher, and thereby calls the idea of the [Freudian] dream-work or censorship into question. It shows that much dream content is coherent, understandable, and readily related to waking concerns. The main "bizarreness" in dreams is sudden scene changes (Sutton, Rittenhouse, Pace-Schott, Stickgold, & Hobson, 1994), which is not usually thought of as a product of the dream-work. These findings still leave a significant amount of dream content to explain ... Whatever the exact amount of remaining dream content that is or is not meaningless, however, the important point for now is that the burden of proof is on those who claim hidden meaning to demonstrate their hypothesis with systematic empirical evidence. (Domhoff 2001, 10-11)

To the empiricists, dream content is not viewed as particularly symbolic, but is instead viewed as often direct and mundane. These are important concepts when studying SRFOs because they suggest that if one thinks about sex or experiences sexual arousal while awake, one is more likely to dream about sex while asleep. Conversely, if one does not think about, or have experience with arousal, sex, or orgasm

138

while awake, one probably would *not* have experience with arousal, sex, or orgasm while asleep.

3. The Neurophysiologists

This next major classification includes the neurophysiologists and sleep researchers who have tended to view dream production as a brain/biology-driven process. In the extreme version of this perspective, epitomized by the Hobson-McCarley "activation-synthesis theory" (1977), the dream contents are essentially "noise," rather random, incidental, and motivationally neutral as part of a larger maintenance function. Nonetheless, learning, insight, problem-solving and creativity might sometimes result. Hobson and McCarley's significant contribution was in identifying the neural pathways which are activated during REM. But for them, initially, dreaming was a mindless activity totally driven by the pons (brainstem).

Subsequent research by Mark Solms (1997), studying the neural network for dreaming using 361 patients with various kinds of brain lesions, showed that some people with pons lesions still dream, and some do not.

> The parts of the brain that are crucial for REM are the pons, which is located in the brainstem near the nape of the neck. The parts of the brain that are crucial for dreaming, by contrast, are situated exclusively in the higher parts of the brain, in two specific locations within the cerebral hemispheres themselves....The first of these location is in the deep matter of the frontal lobes of the brain, just above the eyes (Solms, 1997). This part of the frontal lobes contains a large fibre-

pathway, which transmits a chemical called 'dopamine' from the middle of the brain to the higher parts of the brain. Damage to this pathway renders dreaming impossible but it leaves the REM cycle completely unaffected (Jus et al. 1973). This suggests that dreaming is generated by a different mechanism than the one that generates REM sleep...Chemical stimulation of this dopamine pathway (with drugs like L-DOPA) lead to a massive increase in the frequency and vividness of dreams with out it having any effect on the frequency and intensity of REM sleep. (Solms 1999).

In the last chapter I discussed how dopamine is now viewed as the chemical of pleasure, motivation, addiction, and happiness. Solms' discovery that dopamine and dopamine pathways are necessary for the experience of dreaming and awareness of dreams is important because it allows a role for *motivation*, and *cognition or awareness* in dreaming that Hobson's theory does not. (Hobson subsequently modified his theory.)

Overall, this observation has led to more collaboration between the Freudians, empiricists, and the neurophysiologists. Due to a wide array of new brain imaging technology, it has also led to further investigation of many chemical neurotransmitters in possibly highlighting or tagging certain pre-sleep activities or content for further exploration in dreaming (Gottesmann 1999). How does it happen that pre-sleep emotional involvement often seems to lead to specific content in dreams? In addition to dopamine, the role of acetylcholine has been studied (Schredl and Hoffman 2003). There have been multiple studies of the hypothalamus-pituitary-adrenal (HPA) system in this regard, again suggesting a role for cortisol.

In waking states cortisol increases awareness or vigilance, and it probably plays a role in remembering dreams as well as waking life events. Direct administration of cortisol stimulates greater production of Human Growth Hormone during NREM (especially for men) in those who are depressed (Schmid et al. 2008). Historically, prolonged sleep and rest have been used to treat or re-balance cortisol depletions due to prolonged stress. As mentioned in the previous chapter, the higher pre-awakening cortisol levels during REM seem to allow healthy humans to consolidate new learnings and find resolution or creative problem solutions (Kluger 2012). Cortisol levels might even facilitate SRFOs as a creative problem-solving strategy for restoring system homeostasis. Ultimately sleep cortisol might help us understand better why both anxiety and sexual arousal are correlated with SRFOs.

4. The Consciousness Researchers

Our discussion of dream theories would not be complete without including the consciousness researchers. These really have been the dominant theories throughout human history, essentially highlighting the opportunities which dreaming provides for consciousness expansion, extending awareness into new dimensions of reality and Self, providing a higher, larger, more spiritual perspective. Among this group, dreams are viewed as doorways to the Divine, offering access to the unified field of consciousness and thus allowing experience beyond the limitations of an embodied personality. From this perspective, precognition, telepathy, revelation and communication with a variety of life expressions become natural. These potential opportunities often motivate those who desire to cultivate *lucid dreaming* abilities, which will be discussed shortly.

In recent history, this perspective is often associated with Charles Tart, whose first book, Altered States of Consciousness (1969), became a classic from which the field of Transpersonal Psychology emerged. During the 1960s, Tart conducted numerous studies on the use of hypnosis to influence dream activity, which led to other studies suggestive of out-of-body experiences. Interestingly though, Freud, Jung and Stekel all strongly "asserted the existence of paranormal dreams" (Van de Castle 1995, 405). In 1920, Wilhelm Stekel (a significant contributor to Freud's understanding of symbology, and a major contributor to the field of sexology as well) actually published a book on telepathic dreaming called Der Telepathische Traum (Stekel 1920). Montague Ullman and Stanley Krippner conducted a famous study of telepathic dreaming at Maimonides Hospital in Brooklyn during the 1960s, which they described in their 1973 book Dream Telepathy (Ullman, Krippner, and Vaughan 1973).

While this school of thought is listed last, it is actually the oldest by far. Even before the early Greeks went to the temple to dream, humans sought guidance and contact with the Divine through their dreams. The fact that so many dream stories are included in the Bible is testimony to this fact (King 2006, 98-99).

SEX DREAMS - CONTENT

Although Kinsey presented summary statistics regarding content of the sexual dreams reported by his respondents, he did not feel that this contributed anything new to the study of dream symbolism. His statistics are a bit confusing since, over a lifetime, individual people have many different kinds of dreams. While between 85% to 90% of his sexual dreamers reported having had heterosexual dreams (with 30 to 39% reporting at least one occasion of actual coitus), smaller percentages reported a wider range of sexual dream behaviors including homosexual and sado-masochistic contacts, sex with animals, rape, pregnancy and childbirth. Kinsey did note that many of his sexual dreamers seemed to derive "considerable pleasure from vicariously participating" in these dreams, and compared to men, women were more likely to worry less about their sex dreams and simply accept them as pleasurable (Kinsey et al. 1953, 213-14).

Nonetheless, dream researcher Gayle Delaney (1994) cautions that sexual dreams are significantly different than the sexual fantasies which we can intentionally conjure. Often, sexual dreams are not erotically stimulating. They can have very jumbled plots which are frustrating and/or unpleasant. Whereas rape fantasies are often experienced as pleasurable, rape dreams are not. Other unpleasant sex dreams often include sex with family members, embarrassing situations, violence, being interrupted or "caught." Unpleasant sex dreams usually do not result in orgasm.

Perhaps the most important part of Kinsey's data was the finding that while sex dreams "are often a reflection of experience which the individual has actually had; some 13 percent of the females . . . had had sex dreams which went beyond their actual experience"(Kinsey et al. 1953, 214). The Wells (1986) study found that "dreams were not a significant predictor of nocturnal orgasmic occurrence;" however, "61% reported that their sexual dreams sometimes or always went beyond actual experiences" (Wells 1986, 436). I did not ask

143

about this in my current survey. However, the fact that so many respondents experienced their first orgasms and only orgasms through SRFOs (See Chapter Five) suggests that dream content went beyond experience. (On the other hand, as noted previously, these might have occurred without erotic dreams or any dreams at all.) In addition, many survey respondents voluntarily described dream scenarios which went beyond experience. I think this highlights the natural creativity and learning potential of brain activity during the REM dream state.

There have been numerous studies of the dream content of women during pregnancy. Overall, dream content during pregnancy can be sorted by trimesters, with self-care issues taking prominence during the first trimester; role and relationship issues dominating the second trimester; and the new child dominating the third trimester (Pass 1996).

In 1964, Van de Castle (1971) conducted a content analysis of 450 dreams of female nursing students as they related to different phases of the menstrual cycle. It is interesting to note that while sex dreams occur more frequently during the preovulatory phase, sexual arousal and SRFOs might be more common during the postovulatory, premenstrual phase as noted in Chapter Nine, Table Ten. This again confirms that sex dreams alone are not strongly predictive of SRFOs, as found in the Wells (1986) study cited above. The big exception to this is the case of Lucid Dreaming. Before beginning that discussion, I am going to include a few dream reports from survey respondents.

On another note my dreams are often not sexual at all when I have orgasms, and if they are sexual they are somewhat uncomfortable,

144

such as homosexual. And when I do have dreams of normal sex with my partner I never have an orgasm. I rarely have orgasms when I have sexual contact with a male in my dreams, but if I do it's never my partner and always makes me feel really guilty and uncomfortable when I wake up. (age 19)

I'm a 19 year old female and for the past 4 years I've been having vivid dreams of myself having toe curling orgasms. They are so real, I believe it is really happening. It's usually when I dream of intercourse with a man, though I am a lesbian. (age 19)

A lot of the time there is no visually stimulating sexual content in my dreams, sometimes I am masturbating and sometimes I just move close to a person or press up against someone or something and I have an orgasm. (age 22)

When this happens [SRFOs] it is always hand in hand with an erotic dream, usually dreaming about masturbation and or public sexuality. (age 22)

I have always identified as heterosexual, but most of these dreams are of myself and another woman rather than my husband. (age 22)

Most of them have been dreams about a vibrator or a toy that has s made me orgasm, not men. (age 23)

I think you should ask about sexual orientation and the content of the dream that leads to orgasm. I am a bisexual woman, but I have only had sexual encounters with men (in real life). However, women are almost always the focus of my sexual dreams. I tend to fantasize about women more. Also much of the time I reach orgasm in dreams is from masturbation in the dream. I often become lucid while dreaming during naps, and this often leads to touching and/or masturbation. I always expect to wake up touching myself, but no! (age 24)

I usually remember the dream I'd been having immediately prior to the orgasm (which always wakes me up) and it is usually just beginning to become sexual when I immediately begin having the orgasm. I do not become aroused prior to the orgasm, but rather immediately upon the dream even becoming slightly sexual I have the SRFO. I have also experienced arousing sexual dreams where I did not have an SRFO. (age 26)

I think this is an exciting topic. All the orgasm dreams I have had have been slightly erotic, but I am always by myself. For example – when I was 22 – my first orgasm dream occurred after I had parted with an ex. (age 31)

My first sleep-related orgasm was in high school. I recall dreaming about Jim Morrison and quite curiously, Vince Lombardi. It was weird, but I recalled the dream vividly and the orgasm. For a short time afterward, I had a 'crush' on Vince. I've never been bothered or worried about these dreams, only glad to have them once in a while. (age 35)

Some of the dreams involve sensuality, sometimes with females but not sexual activity. On the other hand dreams about men are very explicit (sexual). (age 35)

Most of my sexual dreams are about having sex with another woman. I'm heterosexual, but I wonder if I'd be bisexual had I grown up in a more permissive society. (age 36)

My orgasms always occur after having a vivid sex-themed dream, either involving intercourse with someone or through masturbation. The ones achieved through masturbation have consistently resulted from dreams where I dreamed I had a penis rather than a clitoris. My most recent one was just this morning and was related to a video I had watched last week of a woman with a very enlarged clitoris who was able to bring herself to climax by manipulating her clitoris in much the same way a man would do with his penis. In my dream, I began by rubbing my clitoris as usual, but then it started to grow bigger and bigger until it was the size of an average penis. (age 36)

After hitting my 40th birthday, and having a rocky relationship with my husband, he became aware of my increased nocturnal orgasms 4-5 night. I do have many dreams and mostly I remember them. But I am not aware of any dream related to these orgasms. My husband became very angry and suspicious, because he thought I was dreaming of a lover. (age 42)

The variation in content of the sexual dreams is very interesting to me. I would say about half of the time I am dreaming about masturbating and the other half am engaging in sexual activity with others. And that activity can vary from same sex to fetish type dreams to oral sex to intercourse. There does not seem to be a pattern. (age 44)

My dreams may have sexual content or not when I have sleeping orgasms and I do awake during the orgasm. Sometimes the dream is very asexual (I may be talking on a pay phone) and other times I am with a man or woman. (age 45)

I have erotic dreams fairly frequently, and at some point these started to result in sleep orgasms. This used to surprise me awake and the orgasm did not complete, however I gradually managed to control my response and allow the orgasm to complete before waking up. The most frequent times they will happen are if I have a sexual fantasy before falling asleep but do not masturbate. In other words I fall asleep with some minor sexual arousal. I have had these types of dreams both with and without an ongoing sex life with a partner. I would say I am normally easily aroused to orgasm by a partner - but without a partner I do not become intensely horny very often and only masturbate about 1 or 2 times a month. (age 48)

Usual dreams are around being in water. Sitting in a hot tub, taking a shower. Typically I am alone. Occasionally, there is someone I do not recognize, who is attractive to me. Typically this is someone of the opposite sex, rarely, it is someone of the same sex. (age 54)

LUCIDITY AND VOLITION

This is another topic that was not addressed by Kinsey since Lucid Dreaming was not popularly recognized at that time. My survey results regarding lucid dreaming were initially surprising to me, and yet, upon reflection make perfect sense. Before getting into my survey, I want to excerpt some information from my first book to clarify the distinctions between lucid dreaming and regular dreaming.

Background

Excerpts from my first book:

Lucid dreaming has been described in literature at least since St. Augustine in 415 A.D., and has been part of the spiritual training in the Tibetan Buddhist and Islamic traditions, as well as the spiritual training of many more primitive cultures, including Native Americans. In recent decades it has become a popular tool in Western spiritual and consciousness explorations. The term is attributed to Dutch psychiatrist Frederik Van Eeden who presented a paper in 1913 at the Society for Psychical Research. He used this term to describe dreams in which he was aware that he was dreaming, had full recollection of his day life, and "could act voluntarily" within the dream (Van de Castle 1994, 440-1).

Normally, this latter quality of volition is an essential element in the definition of lucid dreaming. However, some dream therapists, like Delaney (1994) and Holloway (2001), use this term to mean simply that "you are aware of the fact that you are dreaming while you are asleep having the dream" (Delaney 1994, 26). This is an important distinction, and for purposes of this discussion, the element of volition will be assumed.

Aside from volition, "lucid dreams are often distinguished by the greatly enhanced sensory awareness that appears in them" (Van de Castle 1994, 443). At times, the sensory awareness is so great that lucid dreamers throughout history have often designated this state as another reality. Stephen LaBerge presents a highly useful discussion of this topic in Chapter Nine of his groundbreaking 1985 book, Lucid Dreaming. A result of this condition is that, "Women sometimes have quite vivid sexual dreams in connection with nocturnal orgasms, so much so that on occasion the dreamer may believe she has actually had sex" (Adams 1981).

Lucid dreaming was first demonstrated in a British sleep lab (Hull University) in 1975, and in Stanford University Sleep Lab by Stephen LaBerge in 1980 (under guidance from Dement). It took awhile for either study to be accepted for publishing. In 1981, LaBerge presented four papers on lucid dreaming at the Association for the Psychophysiological Study of Sleep meeting in Massachusetts. Since then, LaBerge has conducted much research through the Lucidity Institute, and published extensively. Today there are many books about lucid dreaming, by many authors. Typically these books also teach techniques for cultivating lucid dreaming skills (Van de Castle 1994, 444-448).

LaBerge's studies require that subjects in a sleep lab, attached to various physiological monitoring devices, provide a particular ocular signal (side to side eye movements) every ten seconds to indicate when they are aware that they are dreaming. Obviously this requires awareness and volition.

The most exciting and satisfying part of lucid dreaming comes from the dreamer's ability to influence the course of the dream events. Influence does not mean total control; however, the ability to participate in an interactive manner leads to interesting experiences and awareness.

Delaney comments that many of her clients and students report that "a number of their orgasmic dreams are lucid ones" (Delaney 1994, 26). Patricia Garfield, author of Creative Dreaming (1974) and Pathway to Ecstasy (1979) writes that:

> *When you become lucid you can do anything in your dream. You can fly anywhere you wish, experience love-making with the partner of your choice, converse with friends long dead or people unknown to you; you can see any place in the world you choose, experience all levels of positive emotions, receive answers to questions that plague you, observe creative products, and in general, use the full resource of the material stored in your mind. You can learn to become conscious during your dreams. (Garfield 1974, 143)*

To date, the only reported incidence of female orgasm during sleep in a sleep lab occurred during a lucid dreaming study conducted by LaBerge in 1983. During the study, the subject signaled with eye movements when she became lucid. She then gave the agreed-upon signal when she initiated sexual activity. This resulted in a fifteen-second orgasm epoch during the REM period of sleep, confirmed by physiological measurements (LaBerge, Greenleaf, and Kedzierski 1983).

Patricia Garfield was one of the first writers to highlight the potential for orgasmic ecstasy during lucid dreaming. Based on the Solms discoveries, we now know that lucidity in dreams requires high dopamine levels to begin with, and the brain wave patterns are more similar to orgasmic states.

> My present hypothesis is this: *Orgasm is a natural part of lucid dreaming.* My own experience convinces me that conscious dreaming *is* orgasmic. Too many of my students have reported similar ecstatic experiences during lucid dreams to attribute the phenomena to my individual peculiarity. There is a kind of mystic experience involved . . . I believe it quite possible that in lucid dreaming we are stimulating an area of the brain, or a chain of responses, that is associated with ecstatic states of all sorts. Sensations of flying, sexual heights, acute pleasurable awareness, and a sense of oneness are all natural outcomes of a prolonged lucid dream.
>
> In my early experiences of conscious dreaming I woke immediately prior to, during, or after orgasm. Now I've learned to stay within that special space moments longer and explore it further. (Garfield 1979, 44-45)

Interestingly, LaBerge states that women report more orgasms from dreams than do men (LaBerge and Rheingold 1990, 26). However, he distinguishes between male orgasms and *wet dreams* (which often are not accompanied by dreams). LaBerge even suggested that lucid dreaming might be an ideal milieu for treatment of female sexual dysfunctions.

> There are both psychological and physiological reasons why the lucid dreaming state tends to be a hotbed of sexual activity. In terms of physiology, our research at Stanford has established that lucid dreaming occurs during a highly activated phase of REM sleep, associated, as a result, with increased vaginal blood flow or penile erections. These physiological factors coupled with the fact that lucid dreamers are freed from all social restraint ought to make lucid dream sex a frequent experience. These findings imply that lucid dreaming could become a new tool for sex therapists, and new hope for those who suffer from some forms of psychosexual dysfunction . . . Like many new ideas . . . this is untested and ripe for research. (LaBerge and Rheingold 1990, 171)

Lucid dreaming occurs quite naturally for many people, especially in childhood. Remember, we spend a higher percentage of sleep in REM during childhood (See illustration 3). Lucid dreaming begins to decrease around age 10 to 12 (Armstrong-Hickey 1991, 250-54) when waking brain wave frequencies shift into a higher range (beta frequencies) and puberty begins. Nonetheless, it is fairly easy to re-learn this ability through a variety of techniques including hypnosis (Dane and Van de Castle 1991), self-hypnosis, autosuggestion, brain-wave training, and meditation techniques, especially among women (Gackenbach 1990). Many people report their first adult lucid dreaming experiences after simply hearing about it and forming an intention to develop it.

On the basis of various studies she had conducted, in 1989, dream researcher Jayne Gackenbach estimated that:

> About 58% of the population have experienced a lucid dream at least once in their lifetime, while about 21% report it with some frequency (one or more per month). Additionally, 13% of dreams recalled on the morning after and recorded in dream diaries are likely to be lucid. (Gackenbach and Bosveld 1989, 91-92)

My survey respondents reported a somewhat higher rate.

Survey Responses (n=200)

10. Do you ever have lucid dreams, in which you are aware you are dreaming and able to influence the content of the dream?
      Yes: 79%   No: 21%

If yes, how often:
    21.5% Less than 10 times in life
    32.5% Several times each year
      15% Several times each month
       9% At least once each week
       1% No estimate

Table 16 – Incidence and Frequency of Lucid Dreaming

Lucidity and SRFOs

Based on research from my dissertation, I hypothesized that SRFOs would be more common among lucid dreamers. Seventy-nine percent of my total group of respondents reported that they had experienced lucid dreams. Of those who had never experienced a lucid dream,

71% had experienced a sleep-related orgasm. Among the lucid dreamers, 91% reported that they had experienced a sleep-related orgasm. So this hypothesis was supported.

My surprise came when I asked the sleep orgasm experiencers if they thought SRFOs were more common with lucid dreams. Based on the Garfield and LaBerge comments above, one would think so. Interestingly, my SRFO experiencers did not agree. Only 28% said they thought SRFOs were more common with lucid dreams.

This original figure included SRFO experiencers who do not experience lucid dreams. However, when I deleted SRFO experiencers who do not experience lucid dreams, the percentages were only slightly different. Only 33.3% of SRFO experiencers who also experience lucid dreams (n=144) thought that SRFOs were more common with lucid dreams.

Survey Responses (n=174)
17h. In your experience, are these sleep-related orgasms more common with lucid dreams (dreams in which you are aware that you are dreaming and can exercise some direction) than non-lucid dreams?
Yes: 28%   No: 69%   No opinion: 3%

Table 17 – Relationship between SRFOs and Lucid Dreams

There were two primary explanations for this. Some survey respondents reported that they carefully direct themselves away from anything sexual while in the lucid dream state because they want to continue other kinds of explorations, and they have learned that sexual feelings will usually wake them up and end their adventures. The more

155

common explanation from respondents was that when they become lucid, the same kinds of sexual inhibitions that occur in wakefulness often prevent an orgasmic response. For example, in a lucid dream state one might not think it is acceptable to have sex with a restaurant waiter, chemistry professor, same-sex friend, or total stranger while among a crowd of on-lookers, or in the other kinds of bizarre scenarios which dreams present. In some cases, one might not think it is acceptable to have sex in a dream at all. In a non-lucid dream, the dreamer does not have control of the situation and has to go along with the plot.

In both lucid and non-lucid dreams, arousal and orgasm seem to happen extremely quickly relative to waking sexual experiences. (See Chapter Seven) Although lucidity allows one to slow things down a bit, the speed often creates a quality of surprise nonetheless. However, the experience of time is significantly distorted in dream states, and without external measurement, it is difficult to say how much time has actually elapsed.

Despite possible inhibitions, some of the lucid dreamers in my survey felt free to enjoy the sexual freedoms and experiences of the lucid dream state.

> I know they are happening, my ability to lucid dream kicks into play, and I encourage the orgasm, and hold back so much until I finally let go and it's unbearably wonderful. I am a lesbian but I will generally have these orgasms in my dreams with my ex who is a man. It's not always him though. I've never had this type of dream about a woman. I can be in the middle of an orgasm dream and my mind will know I'm having one and I will purposely choose not to wake up. I dream of achieving this amazing

feeling when I have sex in the physical world, but not close enough, not like the dreams. (age 19)

I also started practicing lucid dreaming when I was around 15. I can usually make decisions in my dreams, but I hardly ever fully realize that I'm dreaming. And when I do, I wake up soon after. (age 20)

Sometimes I know I'm dreaming but still not able to direct the dream in the way I want it to go. (age 27)

I have always been able to control my dreams, even as a child. I can wake up from a sexual dream and go back to sleep and direct my mind back into the dream I was experiencing prior to waking or create a new dream if I like. I have become very good at balancing between unconsciousness and consciousness to purposely achieve orgasms while sleeping. (age 28)

I can do whatever I want in my dreams and it is nobody's business. I am very open about sexuality. (age 28)

My orgasm dreams include a gamut of partners, situations, and emotions. This morning I had 3 separate dreams, which prompted researching online and finding you. I have lucid dreams where I simply tell myself to orgasm. I have dreams with women, men, my parents, random people from various parts of my life. The theme of my dreams last night was orgasming from giving the orgasm to the other person. I am intrigued to read your initial findings and hope these answers contribute in a meaningful way. (age 28)

I only have the orgasms while I'm asleep and dreaming. If I wake up during the dream I am not physically aroused at all. If I start to become lucid the arousal diminishes and is completely gone by the time I wake up. However, after having the orgasm I wake up. By waking up in the middle of the dream I discovered that I am not touching myself in anyway. (age 34)

But I do find that when I am having a lucid sex dream, I will purposefully guide the dream to bring me to orgasm. This is what I find the most fascinating about the whole thing. I am a very sexual person and love being so. (age 44)

Chapter 11

Will I Ever Experience an Orgasm While I'm Awake?

In most cases, the transition to waking orgasms happens quite naturally due to the ordinary developmental experiences of life: new relationships, , new information, experimentation, etc. However, one of the most surprising statistics from my survey is the number of women, many married, who experienced their first orgasm as an SRFO, and report that **this is the only kind of orgasm that they have *ever* experienced.** In other words, they have never experienced an orgasm while fully awake, either with a partner or through masturbation. Currently, slightly over 10 percent of my experiencers fall into this category. Most are under age 40, although a few range much higher in age.

Here's a sample of comments from respondents:

> I only have orgasms in my sleep! Kind of makes me worried that I will never be able to enjoy them when I am awake. They happened to me when I was younger but I didn't know what they were. How can I achieve these orgasms when I am awake? (age 20)

> I have only had an orgasm during dreams [...] I am afraid that I will never have an orgasm while awake...and I don't seem to find many men (or women, I'm not gay) sexually attractive like I used to [...] I think not being able to orgasm while awake is taking away my

sexuality, since I have no desire to have sex anymore, and the lack of attraction to men. (age 23, married)

How can I take my ability to have orgasms while sleeping, and use it to achieve orgasms with my lover through sex? Is that even possible? I've always read and been told that a certain percentage of women CANNOT orgasm through sex and most likely never will. For me, after having orgasms while sleeping (without any kind of stimulation other than mental) I don't see how I couldn't have an orgasm through sex eventually. (age 28)

Since I was a teenager I've experienced orgasms while I was sleeping. I thought at the time they were the result from reading explicit romance novels. They didn't happen every month but enough in a year's times... It wasn't until I became sexually active and never experienced an orgasm during normal intercourse that I started to believe something is wrong with me. Even oral sex doesn't get me the big "O"; I even tried masturbation and sex toys but nothing works. I know I'm capable of them because I have them in my sleep and they are amazing. (age 27)

One comment I'd like to make is that I've always wondered why it's so relatively easy for me to lucidly orgasm in my dream, obviously with no physical touch at all, while in an awake state I have a VERY hard time reaching orgasm, especially with a partner. I would say that it happens only a small percentage of the time. It makes me think I have a mental block that is

160

lifted when I'm in the dreaming state. (I also cannot orgasm through vaginal penetration while awake, but am able to easily in my dreams.) I want to learn how to merge these two states together so that I'm just as comfortable reaching orgasm in real life as I am in a dream state. (age 26)

I enjoy these sleeping experiences very much, but I find it deeply depressing that I can't seem to climax when awake and entirely cognizant of my surroundings. I'm not aware of having any "hang-ups," and I've tried long baths, vibrators, fantasizing etc. I also have a generous husband who I'm very attracted to and aroused by. But I have never come close to experiencing orgasm awake. (age 33)

I've never been able to reach orgasm during consciousness, either through sex with a partner or through self-stimulation, and up until the point where I started to have them in my sleep I wondered whether there was something physiologically wrong with me. (Clearly this is not the case.) (age 36)

During one point where I was a little awake and talking to my husband...we started having sex and boom...FIRST orgasm ever while I was awake. I was so happy I cried! Since then, I've experienced one small orgasm awake with him. But none of my orgasms while I am awake feel like the amazing, mysterious orgasms I have when I'm dreaming/ sleeping/waking up. Am I broken? ☹ (age 36)

I would really love to be able to orgasm during sex but never in my life have I been able to do this. It is particularly frustrating given I know what I'm missing out on! Thanks. (age 37)

I am frustrated that I cannot have a vaginal orgasm with my partner when I can have these "mental" orgasms on my own. However, I am happy with my sexuality overall.
(age 45)

This is a category that was not addressed by Kinsey. I have read that renowned sex therapist and author Lonnie Barbach (1975), as well as other therapists, have mentioned that some of their clients fall into this category. This topic is now being discussed on some of the internet blogs and health columns. One of the most comprehensive is http://ehealthforum.com/health/topic38773.html. Perhaps, to some degree, this issue arises as a natural result of so many women experiencing SRFOs at young ages as their first orgasms. It is also possible that some women are experiencing waking orgasms, but tend to negate them because they are not as powerful or intense as their SRFOs.

Clinically, this condition fits into the diagnostic classification of Female Orgasmic Disorder, especially if it is causing distress. While a full clinical discussion of this topic is beyond the scope of this book, I want to make a few comments on this condition both to instill hope and provide information.

Overall, with this situation, women who experience SRFOs have a significant advantage over those who have never experienced any kind of orgasm. First of all, SRFO experiencers know that their bodies are capable of orgasm.

So while some of my survey respondents have been worried that SRFOs might indicate that there is something wrong with them, those who have never experienced an orgasm while awake have been delighted because their SRFOs show them that there is nothing wrong with their bodies.

Secondly, women who experience SRFOs have a conscious memory of what arousal and orgasm feel like. This memory provides a valuable reference for transference into waking states.   Thirdly, the SRFO experiences often eventually provide an element of familiarity which leads to greater safety with the waking orgasmic response.

ORGASM TRAINING

In most cases, the incorporation of waking orgasms can be made through a variety of "orgasm training" options ranging from sex therapy (individually, with a partner, or in groups), to books and educational videos. Female orgasm is paradoxical in so many ways. While orgasm is a *reflex*, for women it often also has multiple *learned* components ranging from learning about one's body, to reassessing cultural messages, to feeling safe with high levels of arousal and letting go into the reflex. As theologian and educator Mary Pellauer points out:

> Women cannot take orgasms for granted. Men apparently do so, at least for most of the lifespan. Female orgasm does not come "naturally." We have to *learn* it. While this may also be true of male orgasm, it is emphatically the case for women. What is learned may be learned askew, idiosyncratically, or may be biased by hidden assumptions. Many layers of interpretation swath

experiences of orgasm like veils of shawls. (Pellauer 1993, 150)

Various studies over the years have indicated that a significant percentage of women have NEVER experienced an orgasm while awake or asleep. Reports range from about 8% to 15%. Often this condition is referred to as "anorgasmic." Most sexologists prefer the term "pre-orgasmic" because we know that in many cases, with a little focused attention and training, many of these women can become orgasmic. Of course, it is wise to have a physical examination to determine if there are any medical conditions that need attention. Paradoxically, having orgasm as a goal of sexual contact can actually interfere with experiencing pleasure and orgasm. And yet, without experiencing orgasm at least occasionally, many women lose interest in sexual relations.

I am going to include another excerpt from my first book which addresses this topic:

Since publication of the Masters and Johnson groundbreaking study of Human Sexual Response (1966), and the success of their psychoeducational approach to dealing with Human Sexual Inadequacy (1970), a variety of orgasm training programs have been developed, supplemented by a plethora of self-help books. Aside from Masters and Johnson, LoPiccolo and Lobitz (1972), and Lonnie Barbach (1975) made major contributions to this work. Today, both trained professionals and non-professional entrepreneurs conduct these programs. Formats range from individual or couple sessions in a therapeutic context, to work with groups of women, and groups of couples in more public educational or workshop settings. While some programs emphasize specific philosophies, techniques, or even products, most include the following elements and objectives:

    a. *To provide women with detailed information about female sexual anatomy and encouragement to explore their own bodies.*

    b. *To provide detailed information about the sexual response cycle and typical physiological changes and sensations associated with each stage.*

    c. *To give women permission to think thoughts and have feelings that were previously discouraged, condemned, or even punished.*

    d. *To dispel myths regarding masturbation and orgasm.*

    e. *To encourage women to recognize and value the benefits of masturbation.*

    f. *To create safety and familiarity with personal sensations in response to physical stimulation.*

    g. *To discover personal preferences regarding pleasurable sensations.*

    h. *To develop skill in communicating about personal preferences.*

    i. *To develop familiarity with sensations which trigger the orgasmic reflex.*

    j. *To feel safe "letting go" or surrendering to this reflex.*

k. *To discover and release possible psychological blocks to "letting go."*

l. *To develop safety and pleasurable interpretation of the sensations associated with the orgasmic reflex.*

m. *To feel comfortable experiencing the orgasmic reflex in a variety of settings and conditions; i.e., alone or with a partner.*

There are many specific tips, tools and techniques that can be associated with each of these objectives, but typically they include cognitive behavioral approaches like education, relaxation training, and exploration of arousal patterns through fantasy, as well as physical practice including Kegel exercises, sensate focus exercises, and directed masturbation (DM). As with many learned behaviors, practice makes perfect. "Sex is actually less instinctive in the human being. Like any other skill, it needs to be learned and practiced" (Barbach 1975, 6). As noted earlier, the more orgasms a woman has, the more she can have, and the easier and more pleasurable they are.

> It is precisely because orgasm is a learned response that therapy programs can successfully treat many sexual dysfunctions. Women who have never had an orgasm, for instance, can learn about their bodies' response to various types of stimulation and increase their ability to have orgasms" (Reinisch 1990, 86).

Masturbation

In my dissertation I included a lengthy section on masturbation with a lot of statistics, which I will not repeat here. I do want to emphasize, though, that research over the past forty years or so indicates that masturbation, especially with a vibrator, is the MOST effective tool for assisting women to become orgasmic in waking states. Young women are often not able to masturbate to orgasm in their beginning attempts, so it is not as self-reinforcing as it initially might be for men. It requires some persistence and experimentation. Often young women give up and simply seek coitus to experience the emotional bonding even without physical release/satisfaction. While there is often hope that partnered sex will one day lead to the Big O, when it does not, sometimes women start to lose interest in sex in general.

Masturbation provides a wonderful opportunity to learn about orgasm and sexual responsiveness; and most women do eventually discover their orgasmic abilities without formal therapy or training. "Self pleasuring" tends to become more popular with women as they get older, as they become better educated, and as they become more successful at experiencing orgasm. As noted earlier, once learned, masturbation is often the most reliable opportunity for orgasm in a woman's life (Hite, 1976).

In addition, the women who masturbate most, also experience orgasm most frequently during partnered sex. This is contrary to what many people think, and contrary to how most men experience orgasm. Again, for women, practice makes perfect! And as mentioned in an earlier chapter, women tend to experience orgasm during partnered sex more often as they get older. This is probably testimony to the fact that learning is a life-long experience, and "old dogs" of both sexes really can learn new tricks!

In some cases, knowledge, comfort and confidence with the orgasmic reflex probably contribute to the frequency and ease of SRFOs, just as they do to orgasms during masturbation and partnered sex. This is probably why Kinsey found that masturbation was correlated with SRFOs. This relationship is quite different than the current understanding regarding male nocturnal emissions. Young men are sometimes advised to masturbate before sleep as a way to prevent *wet dreams* (Reinisch 1990, 91). For some women, masturbating before sleep, with or without orgasm, might actually stimulate SRFOs due to lingering physiological arousal.

Fantasy

One of the most interesting aspects of SRFOs is that there is no stimulating physical touch which precedes orgasm. In cases where the SRFOs are preceded by erotic dreams, it is very easy to discern the connection between thoughts and bodily response. Kinsey was of the opinion that SRFOs were primarily the result of "psychologic" factors. While it now appears that there are many other factors at play, including physiological factors, thought and emotion are often part of the SRFO experiences. They are also important parts of stimulating sexual arousal in waking orgasms. For this reason, most women naturally and spontaneously combine physical masturbation with fantasy.

The most common fantasies are simply remembering... remembering your partner's smell or look or a comment...or a time you had great sex. Other common fantasies are simply anticipation about how great it's going to be when you are next with your lover, and what you might do with each other. (Both memory and anticipation will increase dopamine levels.) On the other hand, fantasies often include people and sexual behaviors well beyond what one might incorporate into their actual sexual practices...and well beyond what one might actually desire in real world sex. Both the familiar and the "forbidden" thoughts can lead to physical arousal.

In making the transition to waking sex, it is important for women to become aware of the thoughts and mental images that provoke arousal. Women tend to respond strongly to words. With words, we create our own unique mental images and vicarious emotions. Moving beyond romance novels, female erotica has become a very popular literary genre in recent years. As I write this, the number one bestseller on the "trade paperback" list is *Fifty Shades of Grey* by E.L James, the first book of a trilogy of female erotica emphasizing dominance and submission. Female erotica is a top-selling category for the e-readers. Many books and websites now focus on these titillating stories for women...and keeping up with our cultural changes, there are even "apps" for that!

In addition, newer studies are showing that women do respond, more strongly than was earlier thought, to sexual images as well. Some adult videos today are designed specifically for women. Increasing numbers of women enjoy adult web sites.

In my online survey, 39% of respondents (including both SRFO experiencers and non-experiencers) report that they are sometimes "able to experience orgasm as a result of waking sexual fantasy alone, without any physical stimulation." Studies by Komisurak and Whipple have shown that the physiological responses of women who induce orgasm by "thinking themselves off" are identical to those of physically induced orgasms. While I have not seen statistics related to the general population, this 39% today among my survey respondents contrasts with 2% in Kinsey's 1953 study.

To the degree that "human sexuality is to an unknown extent a creation of the human mind," (Schulz 1984), it is important for women to incorporate fantasy into waking sex in order to make the transition to waking orgasms.

PENIS-VAGINA INTERCOURSE (PVI)

Before leaving this topic, I want to note that even though a woman is able to experience orgasm through masturbation, there is usually a little more learning required to make the shift to orgasm with penis-vagina intercourse (PVI), or even partnered sex with multiple forms of stimulation. Forty-eight percent of my survey respondents reported being able to experience waking orgasm through vaginal stimulation, although PVI was not specified.

In a fairly recent *Psychology Today* article Michael Castleman points out that:

> Vaginal intercourse can feel wonderful: the physical closeness, the emotional intimacy, and for many, the belief that intercourse epitomizes sex. But for women's orgasms, the old in-out is also problematic. The best evidence suggests that only 25 percent of women are consistently orgasmic during intercourse no matter how vigorous or prolonged it is, no matter how loving the relationship, no matter what position the

lovers use, and no matter what the size of the man's penis.

The reason? During intercourse (missionary, doggie, woman-on-top, whatever), the penis does not directly stimulate the clitoris, the organ responsible for women's orgasms. Sexuality experts reassure couples that the woman's inability to experience orgasm during intercourse is (1) very common, (2) no reflection on her sexual responsiveness, (3) no reflection on the man's sexual technique, and (4) no reflection the woman's feelings about the relationship. I agree. (Castleman 2010)

Some techniques, like the Coital Alignment Technique (CAT), emphasize the man's position while "on top" to address clitoral stimulation. Most sex therapists and coaches encourage a variety of manual, oral, and sometimes mechanical stimulation. Dr. Ian Kerner, in his popular book, *She Comes First* (2004), emphasizes oral sex techniques for female stimulation, and quite literally, making sure the woman reaches orgasm first, before PVI. Many therapists recommend that women stimulate themselves manually whenever able; i.e., when on top, or in "doggie style" positions.

The most recent National Survey of Sexual Health and Behavior report concluded that:

Men's orgasm was ... tied specifically PVI. When PVI was absent from the most recent sexual event, men were less likely to orgasm. For women, the path to orgasm appeared to be more variable as they were more (or less) likely to orgasm based on the presence or absence of a range of behaviors. This may reflect the greater variability among women in terms of their orgasmic response or the number of behaviors that many women and their partners engage in as an effort to facilitate female orgasm (Herbenick et al, NSSHB 2010, 359).

This study included a wide range of sexual behaviors and combinations of behaviors including partnered masturbation and anal sex, as well as oral sex and PVI. It did not include the use of "sex toys," also known as "marital aids." Today, many couples regularly incorporate a variety of devices into their sex play. A large selection of sexual lubricants and vibrators are now available at many drug stores and supermarkets. Both "brick and mortar" and online sex toy retailers have focused on becoming more inviting for women. Many devices today have been designed by women, for women, to meet both clinical and recreational needs. In many parts of the United States, home-based sex toy parties are popular, similar to Tupperware parties.

Aside from the physical behaviors, perhaps the biggest challenges to orgasm during partnered sex are psychological. Distractions, worries, and various inhibitions interfere with arousal and orgasm. In addition, women have a tendency to focus on their partners instead of themselves...wondering what the partner is thinking or feeling. It is very important for women to learn to focus on their own desires, sensations, fantasies, and pleasurable interpretations. This is part of the reason why masturbation can be such a valuable training experience...no partner to distract attention.

Women usually need to experience a certain level of trust with their partners in order to shift their focus to themselves. This is why the "sensate focus" exercises popularized by Masters and Johnson are often effective. In sensate focus exercises women learn to simply focus on their own sensation, initially experiencing non-sexual touch by their partner with no demand for sex or orgasm.

A Dutch study using PET scans of female brains during partner-stimulated sex show that during the orgasmic reflex, almost all of the brain becomes "deactivated" except the part of the cerebellum that registers the sensation of being touched or stimulated. Similar to the REM stage of sleep, movement during real female orgasm is not under conscious, voluntary control. Clearly this is an altered state of consciousness (Holstege 2005a). It does require a certain degree of trust to let-go and surrender (to the reflex) in the presence of another.

Ironically, it is the focus on oneself and one's own pleasurable sensations that leads to the expansive experience of orgasm, merging, and energy exchange. Many sex therapists recommend that partners take turns "doing each other." It can be difficult to give and receive at the same time. Different parts of the brain and nervous system are involved. In the past, we used to call this foreplay. In reality, it is THE play. (And yes, sex benefits from a playful attitude and sense of humor, as well as passion and desire.) Every second of sensuous interaction can produce delights. After one is in touch with their own expanding pleasure and sexual arousal, a variety of PVI connections can be made, each offering unique sensations. And sometimes women will orgasm as a synergistic response to their partner's energy and pleasure.

Chapter 12

How Do I Stop or Start Having These

SRFOs?

I receive both of these questions in my emails. There are no absolute answers. Lucid dreaming provides the clearest path for exercising control; however, most SRFOs occur very quickly under conditions in which we are not fully lucid and do not have much control. Nonetheless, clear intentions often lead to desired results in life in general. So, I will make a few suggestions.

STOPPING

Although 77% of my SRFO experiencers reported that they enjoy their SRFOs, quite a few of the young responders found them embarrassing and/or intrusive. This group frequently asked, "How do I make these stop?" While I do think that SRFOs are part of a normal, healthy adjustment to adulthood, and provide valuable learning opportunities, I can also empathize with the concerns of some of my respondents. Long term health and happiness probably depend more on learning to feel safe with these responses, and even enjoy them, rather that stopping them. I have not seen any research regarding stopping SRFOs beyond this survey. Consequently, it is possible that none of these suggestions will work. However, responses from survey respondents have offered some clues.

1. Relax. To the extent that stress or anxiety might trigger these, relaxation exercises could be useful. Physical exercise

also contributes to physical relaxation and balance. Thinking that something might be wrong with you will probably contribute to anxiety. Put that idea aside.

2. Get to know your body better, including the sexual parts. Trust that your body is your friend, and is demonstrating an inherent wisdom on your behalf with its various responses. Over the course of life, it is likely that your beautiful, healthy, female body will surprise you in a variety of ways. Learn to pay attention, listen, and communicate with it.

3. Explore your sexuality while awake, and make peace with it. We are all sexual beings, and your sexuality is natural, healthy, and innocent, despite what others might have told you. Examine your attitudes and seek accurate information.

4. Get adequate sleep so that all of your physical, emotional, and cognitive systems can regenerate on a regular basis.

5. Take birth control pills. To the extent that SRFOs might be hormonally induced, it is likely that birth control pills will stop the mid-month LH surge and some of the fluctuations which influence, or possibly trigger, SRFOs.

6. Talk to others while you are awake. Chances are that at least a few of your friends are experiencing these. Of course, going online to get or share information is often helpful in a variety of ways. Let your bedmates or roommates know that you sometimes experience these sleep orgasms so they will not be surprised or concerned if they observe something. Share this book with your friends.

7. Review your regular drug intake. Although I have not discussed this previously, it is likely that some drugs currently used for Attention Deficit Disorders, especially those with an amphetamine or ephedrine base, can increase dopamine levels and physiological states of sexual arousal (Meston and Heiman 1998). Drugs used during Invitro Fertilization (IVF) treatments can also trigger SRFOs (Chapter 10). On the other hand, most antidepressants are likely to inhibit SRFOs, and are sometimes used in the treatment of NREM sexsomnia. Many drugs are known to influence either dream activity or sexual responsiveness. If you have drug-related concerns, discuss them with your health care provider. It is also likely that some herbal supplements influence SRFOs. In addition, Melatonin, a hormone which is sometimes used to regulate sleep cycles, can induce vivid dreams for some people and cause fluctuations in sex drive in either direction.

8. Choose a dream strategy before going to sleep. Suggest to yourself that if you become lucid or aware in your dreams, you will direct yourself to a particular non-sexual activity. Be gentle and forgiving with yourself if your plans go awry.

9. Develop/keep a sense of humor. Forty-one percent of SRFO experiencers in this survey reported that they found their SRFOs to be amusing or entertaining. Aside from the physical benefits, sometimes the weird juxtaposition of people and events in these dreams can keep you laughing all day!

STARTING

As noted in Table 2, nineteen per cent of the SRFO experiencers in my suvey "actively try to make [themselves] have them." Many others expressed a wish that they might happen more frequently. When I mention this topic in casual conversation, the most common response from those who have never experienced an SRFO is a question about how to start having them. "I want those too!" Personally, I do not really focus on trying to induce them; however, I always appreciate them when they occur. I definitely have appreciated the ones I have had while writing about this topic! I do understand how some people would be curious about things they have not experienced, and I do think that SRFOs have the potential to greatly enhance one's awareness of Self and the entire mind-body system. So, without any judgments about the wisdom of trying to induce these, or guarantees that these ideas will work, here are some suggestions for developing orgasmic responses in sleep.

As mentioned above, our intentions often lead to results. I discussed in Chapter 9 how just thinking about sex can increase sexual arousal, dopamine, and levels of various hormones. It also provides some cognitive material for brain/consciousness to work with in sleep. And as suggested by the work of the dream empiricists, those who think about sex when awake, are more likely to dream about sex while asleep.

In addition, human beings tend to be highly suggestible. A woman once called to let me know how surprised she was to have experienced her first-ever SRFO following a very brief, casual conversation about this topic over lunch the previous day. Another woman told me she lost fifteen pounds from reading my first book as a result of heightened arousal levels, more energy, and spontaneous SRFOs. (Perhaps, awareness of this suggestibility could be one more reason that this topic has not been discussed much in public.) So, a few ideas:

1. Express your sleep/dream intentions before falling asleep. This is often called "dream incubation." Google it. In essence, it means to suggest to yourself in advance the kinds of dream topics and experiences that you would like to have during sleep. Suggest to yourself that you will easily be able to remember and understand your dreams. Of course, if you succeed in having a SRFO, you will probably wake-up and very easily be aware of it.

2. Develop lucid dreaming abilities so that you can choose/create sexually pleasurable dreams experiences if you desire them. There are many books and articles available on this topic, using a variety of techniques including hypnosis. If you notice that inhibitions show up in your lucid dreams, make note of them and address them with yourself while you are awake.

3. Develop your imagination and creativity in general. According to Einstein, "Imagination is more important than knowledge." If you frequently use your imagination while awake, it will probably work better while you are asleep. In addition, you will feel more comfortable in the imaginal realms.

4.. Go to sleep feeling sexually aroused. Read erotic literature and practice generating satisfying sexual fantasies while drifting into sleep.

5. Masturbate before sleep, with or without orgasm. Having an orgasm before sleep might work better than not experiencing one, since women usually have a period of lingering physiological arousal and genital engorgement following orgasm. However, both conditions seem to lead to SRFOs in some cases.

6. Have sex with your partner before sleep, with or without orgasm.

7. If you don't have sex or masturbate, include mild physical exercise before sleep to induce physical arousal and increased blood flow.

8. Go to bed earlier and/or sleep later so that you have a longer REM period before waking up. SRFOs seem to occur more often during the last sleep cycle before morning. Others find that if they wake up and get out of bed for awhile, then go back to sleep, SRFOs are more common.

9. Be in love. Be happy. This keeps your oxytocin and dopamine levels high. When I was young I thought that "being in love" meant that I had to "fall" in love with someone else. Fortunately, I eventually learned that being in love, with all the wonderful feelings we associate with that idea, depends on me alone. Of course, it is always wonderful to share those feelings with others, and over 14% of my survey respondents reported SRFOs to be common at the beginning of a new romantic relationship (Table 10). But the essence of being in love is really an inside job. It begins with the willingness to cultivate a loving relationship with one's Self. Then we can expand it to loving others, loving life,

loving nature, loving beauty, loving creative expression, etc. Some philosophies teach that we *are* love. The same principle applies to happiness. While there are many books and teachings which incorporate these ideas, and many tips about how to produce these results with our choices and behaviors, two recent books which you might find helpful are by Marci Shimoff: *Love for No Reason* (2010), and *Happy for No Reason* (2009).

Chapter 13

Epilogue - Embracing the Inner Goddess

I find myself completing this book during the *Super* Full Moon (biggest and brightest of the year) of May, 2012. In the West, we often link full moons with romance. But in several Eastern spiritual traditions, it is also known as the Wesak full moon, a time of spiritual festivities when contact with the inner planes through dream awareness is said to be easier than usual.

The moon has been associated with feminine sexuality throughout history, and both menstrual cycles and birthing patterns often synchronize with moon cycles. For example, I birthed my son on the night of a *Blue Moon*, the second full moon of that month. To the extent that this book might contribute to a greater understanding of female sexuality, I am taking this full moon as a sign that everything is in perfect timing.

Throughout most of the history of Western civilization, women's sexuality has seemed mysterious to men and women alike. Today we have both the science and the communication tools to change that. We have an opportunity to unravel the myths that bring fear, guilt, self-doubt, and confusion into many lives. We also have the opportunity to embrace the love, joy, ecstasy, power, and wholeness of who and what we are as physical, emotional, mental, and spiritual beings.

And yet, here in the United States we currently find ourselves in the midst of a so-called "War on Women." While some of this is focused on women's pay equality and job opportunity, significant portions are focused on women's health care, sexuality, and reproductive choices with attempts to turn back the clock on cultural and political decisions made decades ago. Those of us who are somewhat older remember well the marches, demonstrations, and consciousness-raising groups of the 1960s and 70s seeking both women's legal rights and sexual freedoms. It seems strange that so much of the current cultural debate is based on ignorance and grossly out-dated assumptions about how life is for women today. Ideally, these legislative attempts will stimulate many younger women to raise their voices and tell their truths. It is up to all of us to keep the conversation real, and provide information where we can.

This book has turned out to be much longer than I anticipated. It has also turned out to be more of a "hybrid" style than I expected. I think I have remained true to my intentions to provide information and reassurance to those who experience sleep-related orgasms, and also stimulate the curiosity of researchers who might want to follow-up on aspects of this topic. My first book lists twenty-seven possible research hypotheses, and I could probably generate a couple dozen more at this point!

In this book, most importantly, I have let women lead, revealing their most intimate experiences, reactions, and opinions. Together, we have lifted the veils. Together we have embraced the Goddess within and let her speak. Thank you.

APPENDIX A

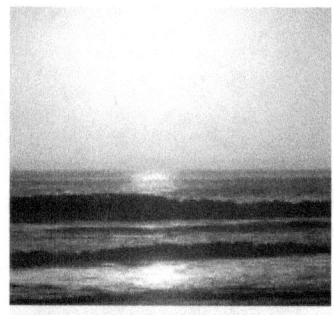

TABLE OF CONTENTS

APPENDIX B

A Research Survey of Sleep-Related Female Orgasms and Sex Dreams©

Conducted by Franceen King, Ph.D.

Dr. Franceen King is a Licensed Mental Health Counselor and Board Certified Clinical Sexologist in private practice near Tampa, Florida. She is also an ordained minister. This survey is being conducted to gather information about several topics that have been neglected in recent sexological research. Information from women of *all* ages and socio-economic backgrounds is needed.

Your participation is completely voluntary and will be greatly appreciated. All information is confidential and will be reported only in anonymous aggregate numbers, or anonymous narrative. Your response to this survey constitutes your informed consent. If you have any questions, please contact me at 813-971-8808, or DrFranceen@aol.com.

You can complete this survey in two different ways: 1) you can copy it into an email addressed to DrFranceen@aol.com, and insert your responses into the email; or 2) you can print this page, write in your responses, and mail it to Dr. Franceen King, 14716 Oak Vine Drive, Lutz, FL 33559.

I hope you find the questions to be interesting and thought provoking. Preliminary results from this survey are discussed here.

Have fun. Thank you for your time and interest.

1. **Current Age**: _____

2. **Race:** _____Caucasian; _____Hispanic; ____African descent; ____Asian descent; _____Native American; _____Other

3. **Marital Status** (Check all that apply): _____Never Married; _____Now Married; _____Previously Married; _____Widowed; _____ Now Living with Partner

4. **Level of Completed Education**: ____Less than High School, ____High School, ____Some college, ____Bachelor Degree, ____Some Graduate School, ____Masters Degree, ____ Doctoral Degree

5. How would you rate your attitudes about sex? Please check.

_____Very conservative,
_____Somewhat conservative
_____Moderate
_____Somewhat liberal
_____Very liberal

6. Have you ever had a dream that you would consider to be overtly sexual or erotic?
_____Yes
_____No

7. Have you ever had a sex dream in which you were having sex with someone else? ____Yes ____No

      If yes, how often:
_____Less than 10 times in life
_____Several times each year
_____Several times each month
_____At least once each week

8. Have you ever had a sex dream in which you witnessed others having sex?
_____Yes ____No

If yes, how often:

_____Less than 10 times in life

_____Several times each year

_____Several times each month

_____At least once each week

9. Have you ever awakened from sleep feeling sexually aroused?

____Yes

____No

If yes, how often:

_____Less than 10 times in life

_____Several times each year

_____Several times each month

_____At least once each week

10.   Do you ever have lucid dreams, in which you are aware you are dreaming and able to influence the content of the dream?

_____Yes

_____No

If yes, how often:

_____Less than 10 times in life

_____Several times each year

_____Several times each month

_____At least once each week

11. Have you ever had a sexual dream that caused you to wake up having a physical orgasm?

_____Yes

_____No

12. Have you ever been awakened from sleep by a physical orgasm without awareness of a preceding dream?

____Yes

____No

13. Have you ever been awakened from sleep by a physical orgasm preceded by a dream without any obvious sexual or erotic content?

_____Yes _____No

14. Prior to this survey, did you know that women sometimes have sleep-related orgasms?

_____Yes

_____No

If yes, how did you first learn about sleep-related orgasms?

_____Sex education class
_____You experienced one
_____A friend told you
_____You read about them in a book or magazine
_____Your mother or older relative told you
_____Other
_____

15. Are you able to experience sexual orgasms when you are awake?

_____Yes, _____No

If yes, indicate all the ways in which you are able to experience orgasm?
_____Through masturbation
_____Through fantasy and masturbation combined
_____Through manual stimulation by a partner
_____Through oral stimulation by a partner
_____Through vaginal penetration by a partner

16. At what age did you experience your first orgasm?

_____Under age 10
_____Between ages 11 and 15
_____Between ages 16 and 20

_____Between 21 and 30
_____Between 31 and 40
_____Between 41 and 50
_____Between 51 and 60
_____Between 61 and 70
_____Over 71

17. If you answered "yes" to #11, #12, or #13, please answer the following questions. Otherwise, please proceed to #18.

17a. Have you experienced a sleep-related orgasm during the past five years?
_____Yes _____No

17b. With or without an accompanying dream, how often have you experienced sleep-related orgasms:

_____Less than 10 times in life
_____Usually about 1 to 5 times each year
_____Usually about 6 to 12 times each year
_____More than once a month
_____More than once a week

17c. At what age do you first remember experiencing a sleep-related orgasm?

_____Under age 10
_____Between ages 11 and 15
_____Between ages 16 and 20
_____Between 21 and 30
_____Between 31 and 40
_____Between 41 and 50
_____Between 51 and 60
_____Between 61 and 70
_____Over 71

17d. During which age periods have sleep-related orgasms been most common for you? (Please rank top three age ranges, as 1= most common; 2= second most common; 3= third most common age period.) Please mark "NA" in the age categories that you have not yet reached.

_____Under age 10
_____Between ages 11 and 15
_____Between ages 16 and 20
_____Between 21 and 30
_____Between 31 and 40
_____Between 41 and 50
_____Between 51 and 60
_____Between 61 and 70
_____Over 71

   17e. Did you experience your first orgasm as a result of a dream or awakening from sleep?
   ____Yes ____No

   17f. During which of the following conditions have sleep-related orgasms
been more frequent for you? Check all that apply.

_____During the premenstrual stage of your monthly cycle
_____During your menstrual flow
_____During the beginning of your monthly cycle, after your menstrual flow
_____During pregnancy. (Check here____ if you have never been pregnant.)
_____During nursing after giving birth
_____During recovery from pregnancy
_____During the beginning of menopausal symptoms
_____After menopause
_____At the beginning of a new romantic relationship
_____During periods of frequent waking orgasms or sexual arousal
_____When between, or without, a sexual relationship
_____After death of spouse or sexual partner
_____During periods of anxiety or worry

_____Other, please describe:

_____

17g. In general, what is your subjective reaction to these sleep-related orgasms? (Check all that apply)

_____You feel worried about them
_____You are confused about them
_____You are embarrassed by them
_____You are curious about why they occur
_____You are afraid of them
_____You enjoy them
_____You used to feel worried, confused, embarrassed or afraid, but you no longer are
_____You find them amusing or entertaining
_____You look forward to them
_____You actively try to make yourself have them

17h. In your experience, are these sleep-related orgasms more common with lucid dreams (dreams in which you are aware that you are dreaming and can exercise some direction) than non-lucid dreams?
_____Yes _____No

18. Have you ever discussed sleep-related orgasms with your physician, gynecologist, or other health care provider?
_____Yes _____No

If yes, briefly describe what they told you.

19. Have you ever discussed sleep-related orgasms with your mental health counselor, psychotherapist, or other psychological advisor?
_____Yes _____No

If yes, briefly describe what they told you.

20. Have you ever discussed sleep-related orgasms with your minister or a spiritual advisor?
____Yes ____No

If yes, briefly describe what they told you.

21. Have you ever experienced orgasm as a result of waking sexual fantasy only (without any physical stimulation)?
___Yes ____No

If yes, how often?

_____Less than 10 times in life
_____Usually about 1 to 5 times each year
_____Usually about 6 to 12 times each year
_____More than once a month
_____More than once a week

22. How would you rate your religiosity?

_____Very religious
_____Moderately religious
_____Only slightly religious
_____Not religious at all

23. With which religion do you most identify:
_____

24. How would you rate your spirituality?

_____Very spiritual
_____Moderately spiritual
_____Only slightly spiritual
_____Not spiritual at all

25. In which kinds of religious and spiritual practices do you normally engage? (Check all that apply.)

_____Personal prayer
_____Group prayer and worship services
_____Private meditation
_____Group meditation
_____Singing
_____Chanting
_____Ecstatic dance or movement
_____Breathwork
_____Guided imagery exercises
_____Spiritual or energy healing
_____Shamanic journeys, or other work in altered states
_____Yoga, tai chi, chi gong, or other mind/body/spirit integration exercises
_____Inspirational reading

26. Please feel free to include any stories, examples, or other comments you would like to make regarding these topics.

Thank you for your participation. Eventually, tallied results will be posted at www.franceenking.com

REFERENCES

Adams, Cecil. 1981. Do women have wet dreams? *The Straight Dope.* Chicago Reader. Accessed 18 March 2005 at www.straightdope.com/classics/al_061.html

Armstrong-Hickey, D. 1991. A validation of lucid dreaming in school age children. *Lucidity* 10, no.1-2: 250-54.

Aserinsky, E., and N. Kleitman. 1953. Regularly occurring periods of eye motility, and concomitant phenomena during sleep. *Science* 118:273-74.

Bancroft, J., J. Loftus, and J.S. Long. 2003. Distress about sex: A national survey of women in heterosexual relationships. *Archives of Sexual Behavior* 32, no. 3:193-208.

Barbach, Lonnie G. 1975. *For yourself: The fulfillment of female sexuality.* Garden City: Doubleday.

Bass, Alan. 1994. Aspects of urethrality in women. *Psychoanalytic Quarterly* 63: 491-517.

Bible (*The Oxford annotated Bible, revised standard edition*). 1962. New York: Oxford University Press.

Calleja, J., R. Carpizo, and J. Berciano. 1988. Orgasmic epilepsy. *Epilepsia* 29, no. 5: 635-9.

Castleman, Michael. 2010. How to boost a woman's chance of orgasm during intercourse. *Psychology Today* accessed 28 January 2012 at www.psychologytoday.com/node/45426

Chalker, Rebecca. 2000. The *Clitoral Truth: The Secret World at Your Fingertips.* New York: Seven Stories Press

Cheyne, J. Allan. 2001. The ominous numinous. *Journal of Consciousness Studies* 8, no. 5-7:133-50.

Cohen, Harvey D., Raymond C. Rosen, and Leonide Goldstein. 1976. Electroencephalographic laterality changes during human sexual orgasm. *Archives of Sexual Behavior* 5, no.3:189-99.

199

Colburn et al. 1996. *Our Stolen Future*. New York: Penguin

Conesa, Jorge. 2000. Geomagnetic, cross-cultural and occupational faces of sleep paralysis: An ecological perspective. *Sleep and Hypnosis* 2:05-111.

Conesa-Sevilla, Jorge. 2004. *Wrestling with ghosts: A personal and scientific account of sleep paralysis.* Pennsylvania: Xlibris Press. Forthcoming 2006. New York: Random House.

Dane, J., and R. Van de Castle. 1991. A comparison of waking instructions and posthypnotic suggestion for lucid dream induction. *Lucidity* 10, no. 1-2:209-14.

Deane, Paul. 2003. *Sex and the paranormal.* London: Vega.

Delaney, Gayle. 1994. Sexual dreams: Why we have them, what they mean. New York: Ballantine Books. Retitled as *Sensual dreaming: How to understand and interpret the erotic content of your dreams.*

Dement, William C. 1974. *Some must watch while some must sleep.* New York: W.W. Norton and Co., Inc.

------. 1992. *Sleepwatchers.* Stanford, CA: Stanford Alumni Asso.

------. 1999. *Sleep paralysis.* Accessed 22 September 2005 at www.stanford.edu/~dement/paralysis.html

Dixon, Jana. 2008. *The Biology of Kundalini* accessed at: http://biologyofkundalini.com/article.php?story=Hormones

Domhoff, G. William. 2001. Why did empirical dream researchers reject Freud? A critique of historical claims by Mark Solms. *Dreaming* 14:3-17. Updates accessed 21 June 2005 at http://psych.ucsc.edu/dreams/Library/domhoff_2004c.html

Exton, M.S., Bindert, A., Kruger, T., Scheller, F, Haratmann, U., Schedlowski, M. 1999. Cardiovascular and endrocrine alterations after masturbation-induced orgasm in women. *Psychosomatic Medicine* 61: 280-289.

Fisher, C, J. Gross, and J. Zuch, 1965. Cycle of penile erections synchronous with dreaming (REM) sleep. *Archives of General Psychiatry* 12:29-45.

Fisher, C., H.D. Cohen, R.C. Schiavi, D. Davis, B. Furman, K. Ward, A. Edwards, and J. Cunningham. 1983. Patterns of female sexual arousal during sleep and waking: Vaginal thermo-conductance studies. *Archives of Sexual Behavior* 12, no. 2:97-122.

Fisher, Seymour. 1989. *Sexual images of the self: The psychology of erotic sensations and illusions.* Hillsdale, NJ: Lawrence Erlbaum Associates.

Finkelstein, Jordan W. et al. 1998. Effects of estrogen or testosterone on self-reported sexual responses and behaviors in hypogonadal adolescents. *Journal of Clinical Endocrinology and Metabolism* 83, no. 7:2281.

Flanagan, Owen. 2000. *Dreaming souls.* New York: Oxford University Press.

Foulkes, D. 1962. Dream reports from different stages of sleep. *Journal of Abnormal and Social Psychology* 65:14-25.

------. 1985. *Dreaming: A cognitive-psychological analysis.* Mahwah, NJ: Erlbaum.

Freud, Sigmund. 1900. *The interpretation of dreams.* In *The basic writings of Sigmund Freud.* 1995. Translated and edited by A. A. Brill. New York: Random House.

------. 1905. *Three contributions to the theory of sex.* In *The basic writings of Sigmund Freud.* 1995. Translated and edited by A. A. Brill. New York: Random House.

Gackenbach, J., and J. Bosveld. 1989. *Control your dreams.* New York: Harper and Row.

Gackenbach, J. 1990. Women and meditators as gifted lucid dreamers. In *Dreamtime and Dreamwork*, ed. S. Krippner, 244-51. Los Angeles: Jeremy Tarcher.

Garfield, Patricia. 1974. *Creative dreaming.* New York: Simon and Schuster.

------. 1979. *Pathway to ecstasy.* New York: Holt, Reinhart & Winston.

Goldey, K.L., van Anders, S.M. 2011. Sexy thoughts: Effects of sexual cognitions on testosterone, cortisol, and arousal in women. *Hormones and Behavior.* doi:10.1016/j.y.hbeh.2010.12.005

Gottesmann, C. 1999. Neurophysiological support of consciousness during waking and sleep. *Progress in Neurobiology* 59, no. 5:469-508.

Guilleminault, C., A. Moscovitch, K. Yuen, and D. Poyares. 2002. Atypical sexual behavior during sleep. *Journal of Psychosomatic Medicine* 64, no. 2:328-36.

Haddon, Genia Pauli. 1993. *Uniting sex, self, & spirit.* Scotland, Connecticut: Plus Publications.

Hamilton, L. D., Rellini, A. H., and Meston, C. M. 2008. Cortisol, sexual arousal, and affect I response to sexual stimuli. *J Sexual Medicine* 5:2111-2118

Hartmann, E. 1966. Dreaming sleep and the menstrual cycle. *Journal of Nervous and Mental Disorders* 143: 406-416.

Heiman, M. 1976. Sleep orgasm in women. *Journal of the American Psychoanalytical Society* 24, no. 5:285-304.

Heiman, Julia, Leslie LoPiccolo, and Joseph LoPiccolo. 1976. *Becoming orgasmic: A sexual growth program for women.* New Jersey: Prentice-Hall.

Henton, C. L. 1976. Nocturnal orgasm in college women: Its relation to dreams and anxiety associated with sexual factors. *The Journal of Genetic Psychology* 129:245-251.

Herbenick, D., Reece, M., Schick, V, Sanders, S.A., Dodge, B., and Fortenberry, D. 2010. An event-level analysis of the sexual characteristics and composition among adults ages 18 to 59: Results from a national probability sample in the United States. *Journal of Sexual Medicine.* 7(suppl 5): 346-361.

Hite, Shere. 1976. *The Hite report.* New York: Macmillan Publishing Co.

------. 1994. *The Hite report on the family.* New York: Grove Press.

Hobson, J. A., and R. McCarley. 1977. The brain as a dream state generator: An activation-synthesis hypothesis of the dream process. *American Journal of Psychiatry* 134:1335-1348.

Hobson, J.A., E.F Pace-Schott, and R. Stickgold. 2000. Dreaming and the brain: Toward a cognitive neuroscience of conscious states. *Behavioral and Brain Sciences* 23: 293-342.

Holloway, Gillian. 2001. *The complete dream book: Discover what your dreams tell about you and your life.* Naperville, IL: Sourcebooks.

Holstege, Gert. 2005(a). Human brain imaging of orgasm in males and females. In *Book of Abstracts.* Conference of the International Academy of Sex Research. Ottawa. July 2005.

------. 2005(b). The orgasmic brain. Interview transcript from *All in the Mind.* Australian Broadcasting Corporation, Radio National. July 9, 2005. Accessed 6 September 2005 at www.abc.net.au/rn/science/mind/stories/s1407052.htm

Holstege, Gert et al., 2005. PET scan results of brain activity during male and female orgasm. Research at Groningen University. Presentation at *European Society of Human Reproduction and Embryology* Conference in Copenhagen. 20 June 2005.

Hufford, David J. 1976. A new approach to 'The Old Hag': The nightmare tradition reexamined. In *American Folk Medicine.* W.D. Hand, ed. Los Angeles: University of California Press.

Janus, Samuel S., and Cynthia L. Janus. 1993. *The Janus report on sexual behavior.* New York: John Wiley & Sons, Inc.

Jemec, Michel. 2007. *Use of lh for generating libido and reaching orgasm in female subjects.* U.S. Patent Application 20070135352

Jus, K., Bouchard, M., Jus, A., Villeneuve, A. & Lachance, R. 1973. Sleep EEG studies in untreated, long-term schizophrenic patients. *Archives of General Psychiatry* 29: 386-390.

Kaplan, Helen Singer. 1974. *The new sex therapy.* New York: Brunner/Mazel.

Kaplan, Helen Singer. 1979. *Disorders of sexual desire*. New York: Brunner/Mazel.

Keesling, Barbara. 1997. *Super Sexual Orgasm*. New York: Harper

Kerner, Ian. 2004. *She Comes First*. New York: Harper-Collins

Khalsa, G.S., Khalsa, J.N.S. 1976. *Study of hormonal changes (Prl, GH, LH) in two kundalini meditations*. Kundalini Research Institute.

King, Franceen. 2011. *Sleep-Related Female Orgasms: A Survey of Biological, Psychological, Sociological, and Cultural Factors*. Lutz, FL: Self-Awareness Publ

Kinsey, Alfred C., Wardell B. Pomeroy, Clyde E. Martin. 1948. *Sexual behavior in the human male*. Philadelphia: W.B. Saunders Company.

Kinsey, Alfred C., Wardell B. Pomeroy, Clyde E. Martin, and Paul H.Gebhard. 1953. *Sexual behavior in the human female*. Philadelphia: W.B. Saunders Company.

Kluger, Jeffrey. 2012. Shhh! Genius at work. *Time* 179, no.16:42-48

Komisaruk, B.R., Whipple, B., Crawford, A., Grimes, S., Liu, W-C., Kalnin, A., and Mosier, K. 2004. Brain activation during vaginocervical self-stimulation and orgasm in women with complete spinal cord injury: fMRI evidence of mediation by the Vagus nerves. *Brain Research, 1024*: 77-88.

Komisaruk, B.R., Whipple, B., Nasserzadeh, S., Beyer-Flores, C. 2010. *The orgasm answer guide*. Baltimore: The Johns-Hopkins University Press.

Korda, Joanna B. et al. 2009. Persistent genital arousal disorder: A case report in a woman with lifelong PGAD where serendipitous administration of varenicline tartrate resulted in symptomatic improvement. *Journal of Sexual Medicine*. 6 (5): 1479-1486.

Kramer, H. and J. Sprenger. 1971, [1486]. *Malleus maleficarum*. English translation by M. Summers and J. Rodker, 1928. Reprinted with 1948 introduction in 1971. New York: Dover Publications.

Kramer, Samuel Noah. 1963. *The Sumerians*. Chicago: University of Chicago Press.

Kremsdorf, Ross B., Lucy J. Palladino, Douglas D. Polenz, and Barbara J. Anista. 1978. Effects of the sex of both interviewer and subject on reported manifest dream content. *Journal of Consulting and Clinical Psychology* 46, no. 5:1166-7.

Kudielka, B.M. and Kirschbaum, C. 2003. Awakening cortisol responses are influenced by health status and awakening time but not by menstrual cycle phase. *Psychoneuroendocrinology* 28:35-47

Kuriansky, Judy. 2002. *The complete idiot's guide to Tantric sex.* Indianapolis: Alpha Books.

LaBerge, S., W. Greenleaf, and B. Kedzierski. 1983. Physiological responses to dreamed sexual activity during lucid REM sleep. *Psychophysiology* 20:454-5.

LaBerge, Stephen. 1985. *Lucid dreaming.* New York: Ballantine.

LaBerge, Stephen, and Howard Rheingold. 1990. *Exploring the world of lucid dreaming.* New York: Ballantine Books.

LaFerla, John J., Anderson, Donald L., and Schalch, Don S. 1978. *Psychoendodrine Response to Sexual Arousal in Human Males.* Psychosomatic Medicine. 40:2

LoPiccolo, Joseph, and Charles Lobitz. 1972. The role of masturbation in the treatment of orgasmic dysfunction. *Archives of Sexual Behavior* 2, no. 2:163-171.

MacDonald, K. and MacDonald, T.M. 2010. The peptide that binds: a systematic review of oxytocin and its prosocial effects in humans. *Harvard Review Psychiatry.* 18: 1-21.

Mah, Kenneth and Yitzchak Binik. 2005. Are orgasms in the mind or the body? Psychosocial versus physiological correlates of orgasmic pleasure and satisfaction. *Journal of Sex and Marital Therapy* 31, no. 3:187-200.

Mangan, M. A. 2004. A phenomenology of problematic sexual behavior occurring in sleep. *Archives of Sexual Behavior* 33, no. 3:287-93.

------. 2005. *Sexomnia Bulletin – April, 2005.* Accessed 23 June 2005 at www.Sleepsex.org

Maslow, Abraham H. 1942. Self-esteem (dominance-feeling) and sexuality in women. *Journal of Social Psychology* 16: 259-294. Reprinted in DeMartino, M.F. ed., 1963. 113-143. *Sexual behavior and personality characteristics.* New York: Citadel Press.

Masters, William H., and Virginia E. Johnson. 1966. *Human sexual response.* Boston: Little, Brown & Co.

------. 1970. *Human sexual inadequacy.* Boston: Little, Brown & Co.

Masters, William H., Virginia E Johnson, Robert C. Kolodny. 1982. *Masters and Johnson on sex and human loving.* Boston: Little Brown & Co.

McNamara, Patrick. 2011. Oxytocin, sleep, and dreams. *Psychology Today.* Accessed on 28 January 2012 at: www.psychologytoday.com/print/72890

Meston, Cindy, and Julia Heiman. 1998. Ephedrine-activated physiological sexual arousal in women. *Archives of General Psychiatry* 55:652-656.

Meston, Cindy, and Penny F. Frohlich. 2003. Love at first fright: Partner salience moderates roller-coaster-induced excitation transfer. *Archives of Sexual Behavior* 32, no. 6:537-544.

Meston, Cindy, Elaine Hull, Roy J. Levin, and Marca Sipski. 2004. Disorders of orgasm in women. *The Journal of Sexual Medicine* 1:66-68.

Michael, Robert T., John H. Gagnon, Edward O. Laumann, and Gina Kolata. 1994. *Sex in America – A definitive survey.* New York: Little, Brown and Company.

Moffitt, T. E., Caspi, A. Belsky, J. & Silva, P. A. 1992. Childhood experience and onset of menarche: A test of a sociobiological model. *Child Development* 63: 47-58.

Montorsi, F, Oettel, M. 2005. Testosterone and sleep related erections an overview. Journal of Sexual Medicine. Nov(6): 771-84.

Morin, Jack. 1995. *The erotic mind.* New York: Harper Collins.

Nepomnaschy, P.A., Altman, R. M., Watterson, R., Co, C., McConnell, D.S., et al. 2011. Cortisol excretion independent of menstrual cycle day? A longitudinal evaluation of first morning urinary specimens. *PLoS ONE* 6(3):e18242.doi:10.1371/journal.pone.0018242

206

NIH (National Institutes of Health). Information about sleep. Teachers guide. Accessed 26 January 2012 at http://science.education.nih.gov/supplements/nih3/sleep/guide/info-sleep.htm

Ogden, Gina. 2006. *The heart and soul of sex: making the ISIS connection.* Boston: Trumpeter

Palace, Eileen M., and Boris. B. Gorzalka. 1990. The enhancing effects of anxiety on arousal in sexually dysfunctional and functional women. *Journal of Abnormal Psychology* 99, no. 4:403-11.

Pass, Cleo Massicotte, 1996. Sleep dreams of women in the childbearing years: A review of research. *Holistic Nursing Practice.* (July): 65-77.

Pellauer, Mary D. 1993. The moral significance of female orgasm: Toward sexual ethics that celebrates women's sexuality. In *Sexuality and the sacred: Sources for theological reflection.* Sandra P. Longfellow and James B. Nelson, eds., 149-168. Louisville, KY: Westminster/John Knox Press.

Persinger, Michael. 1987. *Neuropsychological base of God beliefs.* New York: Praeger.

Purves 2004. *Neuroscience: Third Edition.* Massachusetts, Sinauer Associates, Inc.

Reich, Wilhelm. 1973 [1942] *The function of the orgasm.* (Reprint) New York: Simon & Schuster

Reinisch, June M., with Ruth Beasley. 1990. *The Kinsey Institute new report on sex.* New York: St. Martin's Press.

Robbins, Paul R., Roland H. Tank, and Faraneh Houshi. 1985. Anxiety and dream symbolism. *Journal of Personality* 53, no. 1:17-22.

Robinson, Marnia 2009. *Cupid's Poinsoned Arrow.* Berkeley, CA: North Atlantic Books

Rogers, Gary S., Robert. L. Van de Castle, William S. Evans, and Joseph W. Critelli. 1985. Vaginal pulse amplitude response patterns during erotic conditions and sleep. *Archives of Sexual Behavior* 14, no. 4:327-42.

Ruff, R. L. 1980. Orgasmic epilepsy [letter]. *Neurology* 30, no. 11:1252.

Schmid, D.A., Brunner, H., Lauer, C.J., Rhr, M., Yassouridis, A., Holsboer, F., Friess, E. 2008. Acute cortisol administration increases sleep depth and growth hormone release in patients with major depression. *J Psychiatric Research*: 42(12):991-9

Schredl, M. and F. Hofmann. 2003. Continuity between waking activities and dream activities. *Journal of Conscious Cognition* 12, no. 2:298-308.

Schulz, David A. 1984. *Human sexuality*. Englewood Cliffs, NJ: Prentice Hall.

Shafik, Ahmed, Olfat El Sibai, Ali Shafik, Ismail Ahmed, and Randa M. Mostafa. 2004. Electrovaginogram: Study of the vaginal electric activity and its role in the sexual act and disorders. *Archive of Gynecology and Obstetrics* 269, no. 4:282-286.

Shafik, A., Shafik, A.A., Sibai, O.E., and Shafik, I.A. 2007. Identification of a vaginal pacemaker: An immunohistochemical and morphometric study. *Journal of Obstetrics and Gynaecology*. 27(5): 485-8.

Shapiro, Colin.M., J. Paul. Fedoroff, and Nikola. N. Trajanovic. 1996. Sexual behavior in sleep: A newly described parasomnia. *Sleep Research* 25:367.

Sherfey, Mary Jane. 1972. *The nature and evolution of female sexuality*. New York: Random House.

Shimoff, Marci. 2009. *Happy for No Reason.* New York: Free Press

Shimoff, Marci. 2010. *Love for No Reason*. New York: Free Press

Sipski ML, Alexander CJ, Rosen RC. 2001. Sexual arousal and orgasm in women: effects of spinal cord injury. *Ann Neurol.*,49:35-44.

Solms, Mark. 1997. *The neuropsychology of dreams: A clinico-anatomical study*. Mahwah, NJ: Erlbaum

Solms, Mark. 1999. The interpretation of dreams and the neurosciences. British Psychoanalytical Society. Accessed: 4 March 2012 at http://www.psychoanalysis.org.uk/solms4.htm

Stein, R.A, Oz, M.C., eds. 2004. *Complementary and Alternative Cardiovascular Medicine: Clinical Handbook*. New Jersey: Humana Press
Stekel, Wilhelm. 1920. *Der telepathische traum*. Berlin: Johannes Baum.

Stubbs, Kenneth Ray. 2000. *The essential tantra: a modern guide to sacred sexuality*. New York: Tarcher/Putnam

Sutton, J., C. Rittenhouse, E. Pace-Schott, R. Stickgold, and J. Hobson. 1994. A new approach to dream bizarreness: Graphing continuity and discontinuity of visual attention in narrative reports. *Consciousness and Cognition* 3:61-88.

Talbot, Nicci. 2011. *The libido survey*. Accessed 2 March 2012 at www.inrudehealth.com/features/the-libido-survey.php

Tapia, F., Werboff, J., and Winokur, G. 1958. Recall of some phenomena of sleep: A comparative study of dreams, somnambulism, orgasm, and enuresis in a control and neurotic population. *Journal of Nervous and Mental Disorders* 127:119-23.

Tart C. 1969. *Altered states of consciousness: A book of readings*. New York: Wiley.

Tennov, Dorothy. 1979. *Love and limerence: The experience of being in love*. Chelsea, Michigan: Scarborough House.

Terman, L. M., and M. H. Oden. 1959. *The gifted group at mid-life*. Stanford, California: Stanford University Press.

Tiefer, Leonore. 1995. *Sex is not a natural act and other essays*. Boulder, CO: Westview Press.

The female sexual nervous system. The Clitoris.com http://www.the-clitoris.com/n_html/female_sexual_nervous_system_1.htm

Ullman, M., S. Krippner, and A. Vaughan. 1973. *Dream telepathy*. New York: Macmillan.

Van de Castle, Robert. 1971. *The psychology of dreaming*. Morristown, N.J: General Learning Press.

-------. 1994. *Our dreaming mind*. New York: Ballantine Books.

Wade, Jenny. 2004. *Transcendent sex*. New York: Simon & Schuster.

Wagner, G. (Producer). 1973. *Physiological responses of the sexually stimulated female in the laboratory* (Film). New York: Focus International.

Wells, Barbara L. 1983. Nocturnal orgasms: Females' perceptions of a "normal" sexual experience. *Journal of Sex Education and Therapy* 9:32-38.

-------. 1986. Predictors of female nocturnal orgasms: A multivariate analysis. *Journal of Sex Research* 22:421-37.

Whipple, Beverly, Gina Ogden, and Barry R. Komisaruk. 1992. Physiological correlates of imagery-induced orgasm in women. *Archives of Sexual Behavior* 21, no. 2:121-33.

Whipple, Beverly, and Barry R. Komisaruk. 1985. Elevation of pain threshold by vaginal stimulation in women. *Pain* 21:357-67.

-------. 1988. Analgesia produced in women by genital self-stimulation. *Journal of Sex Research* 24:130-40.

Winokur, G., Guze, S. B., and Pfeiffer, A. B. 1959. Nocturnal orgasm in women: Its relation to psychiatric illness, dreams and developmental and sexual factors. *A.M.A. Archives of General Psychiatry* 1:180-84.

Zillman, D. 1971. Excitation transfer in communication mediated aggressive behavior. *Journal of Experimental Social Psychology* 7:419-434.